Angelo Mosso's

Circulation of Blood in the Human Brain

Angelo Mosso's
Circulation of Blood in the Human Brain

EDITED, WITH COMMENTARY, BY

MARCUS E. RAICHLE, MD

WASHINGTON UNIVERSITY

GORDON M. SHEPHERD, MD, DPHIL

YALE UNIVERSITY

TRANSLATION BY

CHRISTIANE NOCKELS FABBRI, PHD

YALE UNIVERSITY

OXFORD
UNIVERSITY PRESS

OXFORD
UNIVERSITY PRESS

Oxford University Press is a department of the University of Oxford.
It furthers the University's objective of excellence in research, scholarship,
and education by publishing worldwide.

Oxford   New York
Auckland   Cape Town   Dar es Salaam   Hong Kong   Karachi
Kuala Lumpur   Madrid   Melbourne   Mexico City   Nairobi
New Delhi   Shanghai   Taipei   Toronto

With offices in
Argentina   Austria   Brazil   Chile   Czech Republic   France   Greece
Guatemala   Hungary   Italy   Japan   Poland   Portugal   Singapore
South Korea   Switzerland   Thailand   Turkey   Ukraine   Vietnam

Oxford is a registered trademark of Oxford University Press
in the UK and certain other countries.

Published in the United States of America by
Oxford University Press
198 Madison Avenue, New York, NY 10016

Library of Congress Cataloging-in-Publication Data
Mosso, A. (Angelo), 1846–1910, author.
[Sulla circolazione del sangue nel cervello dell'uomo. English]
Angelo Mosso's Circulation of blood in the human brain / edited, with commentary, by
Marcus E. Raichle, Gordon M. Shepherd ; translation by Christiane Nockels Fabbri.
    p. ; cm.
Circulation of blood in the human brain
ISBN 978-0-19-935898-4 (hardback : alk. paper)
I. Raichle, Marcus E., editor, writer of added commentary.   II. Shepherd, Gordon M., 1933– ,
editor, writer of added commentary.   III. Title.   IV. Title: Circulation of blood in the human
brain.
[DNLM: 1. Cerebrovascular Circulation—physiology.   2. Brain—blood supply. WL 302]
QP108.5.C4
612.8'24—dc23
      2014028294

The science of medicine is a rapidly changing field. As new research and clinical experience broaden
our knowledge, changes in treatment and drug therapy occur. The author and publisher of this
work have checked with sources believed to be reliable in their efforts to provide information that
is accurate and complete, and in accordance with the standards accepted at the time of publication.
However, in light of the possibility of human error or changes in the practice of medicine, neither
the author, nor the publisher, nor any other party who has been involved in the preparation or
publication of this work warrants that the information contained herein is in every respect accurate
or complete. Readers are encouraged to confirm the information contained herein with other
reliable sources, and are strongly advised to check the product information sheet provided by the
pharmaceutical company for each drug they plan to administer.

9 8 7 6 5 4 3 2 1
Printed in the United States of America
on acid-free paper

TABLE OF CONTENTS

Brain imaging is one of the most powerful tools in modern research on brain function in health and disease. The dramatic images of different regions of the brain becoming active in response to different behaviors and emotional states reflect changes in the circulation of blood to these regions. Few realize that the origins of this approach go back to around 1880, to a pioneering physiologist who was presented with several individuals whose brains, by trauma or disease, had been exposed to direct observation and who seized the opportunity to obtain the first evidence of changes in the circulation of the blood to the brain being related to changes in human cognitive and emotional behavior. This pioneer was an Italian, Angelo Mosso, who became one of the leading physiologists of his time.

The book summarizing his studies is a masterpiece. Mosso first gives a full background of then-current understanding of brain structure and function. He provides a detailed description of his new method for studying changes in the circulation of the blood. He explains how he realized that he had a unique opportunity in three subjects to apply his method to the circulation of the blood in the brain. The descriptions of his results are classics in the scientific method applied to the most challenging organ of all, the human brain. Mosso concludes with the significance of his findings in the context of what was then known about brain function. Beyond this historical interest, his original study tells a dramatic story that gives insight into the creative process in science, exemplifying Pasteur's axiom that in the field of observation, chance favors the prepared mind.

Mosso's studies were first summarized in a monograph in Italian, followed by a German edition, both of which are still unavailable in English. As two investigators involved in the development of modern brain imaging in humans and in laboratory research, we have felt it important to arrange for the translation of this historic volume. The present work brings long-overdue recognition to Mosso as a founder of modern brain imaging and modern cognitive neuroscience. In Dr. Christiane Nockels Fabbri we found an outstanding translator and are much indebted to her for her meticulous text. As the translation evolved, GMS reviewed it with her in detail from the point of view of what was known about neuroscience during the period of the late 19th century. In turn, MER has examined the entire manuscript from the perspective of the evolution of human brain imaging and cognitive studies.

Mosso's meticulous approach to human physiology is on full display in this volume. The direct observations on the relation of behavior to brain circulation are reported in Chapters 1 through 5, 7, 9, 12, and 13. But he takes pains to support his conclusions in relation to many previous and current investigations of the circulation in general. He thus reports there and in the other chapters his extensive experiments on himself, colleagues, dogs, and rabbits for the effects of the circulation in the arms and body on the changes observed in the brain; the possible influence of respiratory movements on brain circulation; and the effects on brain circulation of pharmacological agents, anemia and hyperemia, and cerebrospinal fluid.

The reader will note the abundant illustrations in the text. The majority, apart from several graphic images of Mosso's subjects and experimental apparatus, are tracings of brain pulsations recorded under a variety of conditions. While these may seem repetitive to modern readers, we nevertheless emphasize that they were some of the earliest published recordings by Mosso's new plethysmograph, an instrument that enabled him to measure and document for the first time objective changes in cerebral blood flow. Careful correlation with the text will enable the reader to appreciate the insights Mosso achieved with each of these recorded measurements.

For further background on Mosso and his many-faceted career, the reader may wish to consult excellent accounts by Cogo et al. (2000), Iadecola (2002), Di Giulio et al. (2006), Zago et al. (2009), and Sandrone et al. (2012). Here we provide a brief orientation to his life within the specific context of his studies of the brain, followed by a Commentary, building on Raichle (2000) and Shepherd (2010), on the subsequent development of modern brain imaging and its current role in understanding brain function in health and disease.

REFERENCES

Cogo A, Ponchia A, Pecchio O, Losano G, Cerretelli P (2000) Italian high altitude laboratories: past and present. High Alt Med Biol 1:137–147.

Di Giulio C, Daniele F, Tipton C (2006) Angelo Mosso and muscular fatigue: 116 years after the first congress of physiologists: IUPS commemoration. Adv Physiol Educ 30:51–57.

Iadecola C (2002) Intrinsic signals and functional brain mapping: caution, blood vessels at work. Cereb Cortex 12:223–224.

Raichle M (2000) A brief history of human functional brain mapping. In: Brain Mapping: The Systems (Toga A, Mazziotta J M, eds), pp 33–75. San Diego: Academic Press.

Sandrone S, Bacigaluppi M, Galloni M, Martino G (2012) Angelo Mosso (1846-1910). J Neurol 259:2513–2514.

Shepherd G (2010) Creating Modern Neuroscience: The Revolutionary 1950s. New York: Oxford University Press.

Zago S, Ferrucci R, Marceglia S, Priori A (2009) The Mosso method for recording brain pulsation: the forerunner of functional neuroimaging. Neuroimage 48:652–656.

BRIEF BIOGRAPHY OF ANGELO MOSSO
AND HIS TIMES

Angelo Mosso (Fig. 1) was born on May 30, 1846, in Chieri, Piedmont, near Turin, in Italy. As a boy he often helped his father, a carpenter, in his work, which gave him practical experience in handling tools and equipment. He was raised in near poverty, which gave him a lifelong commitment to using science to relieve the physical and mental burdens of workers. He studied medicine in the University of Turin Medical School, and upon graduating in 1870 served for 2 years as a military medical officer. To pursue an academic career, he took training under Moritz Schiff in Florence, Carl Ludwig in Leipzig, and Claude Bernard in Paris during the 1870s, which stimulated his interest in the physiology of the vascular system. From Schiff (Haymaker and Schiller, 1970) he learned about the nervous control of the blood vessels that enables them to constrict or dilate in response to local activity in the body. Bernard, too, had studied vasomotor control as part of his characterization of how the body maintains the constancy of its "milieu interieur" (Hoff and Guillemin, 1967).

Ludwig was particularly important for Mosso's training, because he had invented the kymograph in 1846, one of the first mechanical instruments for the quantitative study of bodily processes. This was a blackened paper on a rotating drum, on which a needle inscribed the movements of a physiological experiment, such as the beating of an excised turtle heart or the contraction of a skeletal muscle. (This instrument was still in use, as this writer can attest, complete with blackening the paper over a sooty flame, in student physiological laboratories at Harvard and Oxford in the late 1950s and early 1960s.) Ludwig applied the kymograph to record the varying pressure in blood vessels, regarded as the first objective means of measuring physiological variables. Mosso adopted this approach to measuring volume changes in the kidney and other organs (Di Giulio et al., 2006) and became inspired to apply this "graphical method" to registering objectively physiological changes. During this time Mosso also met other German leaders of the new scientifically based physiology, such as Emil Du Bois Reymond and Ernst von Brucke (reviewed in Shepherd, 1991). To finish his European tour, in Paris he visited Claude Bernard and especially Etienne-Jules Marey, the pioneer of cinematography and scientific measuring approaches such as myography (Di Giulio et al., 2006).

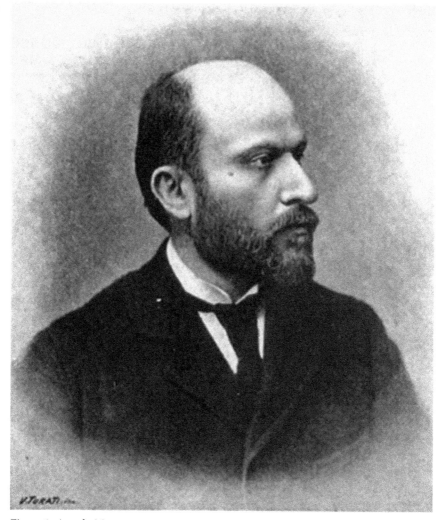

Figure 1 Angelo Mosso

All of these mentors gave Mosso superb training and stimulated his interest in the physiology of the circulation, particularly in methods for registering the changes in blood volume related to the arterial pulse and to muscle contractions in humans. For this work he developed an apparatus to encase the arm in a water-filled cylinder with a water-filled line transmitting the changes in volume during muscular contraction to a recording arm inscribing the movements on a kymograph. This became the Mosso plethysmograph. A later device for measuring fatigue in a contracting muscle was the ergograph.

Upon returning to Turin, Mosso was appointed professor of pharmacology at the age of 30 in 1876, and then professor of physiology in 1879. During this time he pursued the study of blood circulation in the arm using his new plethysmograph, which gave evidence of a high sensitivity of the peripheral circulation to the behavioral state of the subject, especially different degrees of muscle activity, as well as different emotional states such as fear or anger. His first publications were summarized in a book *Diagnosis of the Pulse* in 1879, which came to the attention of, among others, the psychologist William James at Harvard, who wrote:

> The researches of Mosso with the plethysmograph have shown that not only the heart, but the entire circulatory system, forms a sort of sounding-board, which every change of our consciousness, however slight, may make reverberate. Hardly a sensation comes to us without sending waves of alternate constriction and dilatation down the arteries of our arms. (James, 1884)

We will see that James continued to hold Mosso in high regard in assessing his study of brain circulation.

Mosso's study of the brain arose through an unusual opportunity at this early stage in his career. He describes it as follows:

> The technological perfecting of the method of continuous recording of the human pulse in the forearm and in the brain that I had achieved, and the fortunate chance to be able to observe a typical skull defect, allowed me, together with Dr. De Paoli, to perform such an important series of graphic studies of the blood circulation in the human brain that in the present work I shall barely be able to take into account similar studies of other researchers, and am permitted to consider almost exclusively my own observations.[1]

The full context for those remarks will be found in the present book, an extended monograph describing the three patients who were brought to him with disorders of the cranium that exposed the surface of the brain. With his experience in observing vascular pulsations related to muscle activity, he realized that similar pulsations took place in the vasculature of the brain surface that might be related to brain activity. Furthermore, as indicated by James's comment, he was alert to the possible relation between changes in blood flow within the body and changes in behavioral state.

The resulting monograph was published first in Italian. An expanded German edition quickly followed, which is indicative of the general interest in the subject. Translation into German was common, indeed necessary, in the late 19th century, for Germany was the driving force behind the rise of modern science during that period. Our translation into English is therefore from the German version, because this would have been the one most widely read at that time. Subsequently, in 1894, Mosso reported a fourth subject, Luigi Cane, in whom changes of blood flow to the brain were noted to be affected by mental effort and emotion in a manner similar to the observations reported in this volume.

The significance of Mosso's observations for brain imaging is discussed in greater detail in the Commentary. Although Mosso has been largely forgotten until recently, his work in fact had a significant impact on many of his contemporaries. In reviewing these early studies, Zago et al. (2009) note that "Mosso's method was used by numerous Italian and European experimenters to study changes in the brain blood flow during cognitive and emotional experiments, as well as after the administration of drugs" (for over a dozen references to this work, see Zago et al., 2009).

Perhaps the best gauge of the importance of Mosso's work at that time was William James's account of what was then known about the physiology of the brain. We have seen that James, with his interest in both human physiology and psychology, had been following Mosso's work on changes in blood flow related to sensation and consciousness, and this new volume did not escape his attention. In his monumental *The Principles of Psychology*, published in 1890, he built the foundation of human psychology on principles of physiology.

James started with the reflex, as exemplified in the frog, moving to the localization of function in the brain and the phenomena of phrenology, and on to the emerging scientific evidence for physiological localization of the different sensory and motor areas. This was followed by an extensive chapter "On Some General Considerations of Brain-Activity," which included detailed consideration of "the summation of stimuli," "reaction time," "cerebral blood supply," "cerebral thermometry," and "phosphorous and thought." The last item addressed early evidence for chemical reactions that might underlie brain activity. This was based on measuring changes in phosphate in the urine related to mental activity, leading to the catch phrase "The brain secretes thought the way the kidney secretes urine." James dismissed this as a lame analogy, observing that "the materials which the brain pours into the blood (cholinterin, creatin, xanthin, or whatever they may be) are the analogues of the urine and the bile. . . . As far as those matters go, the brain is a ductless gland," an amazingly prescient anticipation of modern brain biochemistry.

In the section on "Cerebral Blood-Supply," James gives testimony to the important new insights that Mosso had provided into the relation between blood supply and cerebral function. We quote this section in full:

The next point to occupy our attention is the changes of circulation which accompany cerebral activity.

All parts of the cortex, when electrically excited, produce alterations both of respiration and circulation. The blood-pressure rises, as a rule, all over the body, no matter where the cortical irritation is applied, though the motor zone is the most sensitive region for the purpose. Elsewhere the current must be strong enough for an epileptic attack to be produced. [2] Slowing and quickening of the heart are also observed, and are independent of the vaso-constrictive phenomenon. Mosso, using his ingenious "plethysmo-graph" as an indicator, discovered that the blood-supply to the arms diminished during intellectual activity, and found furthermore that the arterial tension (as shown by the sphygmograph) was increased in these members (see Fig. 23). So slight an emotion as that produced by the entrance of Professor Ludwig into the laboratory was instantly followed by a shrinkage of the arms.[3] The brain itself is an excessively vascular organ, a sponge full of blood, in fact; and another of Mosso's inventions showed that when less blood went to the arms, more went to the head. The subject to be observed lay on a delicately balanced table which could tip downward either at the head or at the foot if the weight of either end were increased. The moment emotional or intellectual activity began in the subject, down went the balance at the head-end, in consequence of the redistribution of blood in his system. But the best proof of the immediate afflux of blood to the brain during mental activity is due to Mosso's observations on three persons whose brain had been laid bare by lesion of the skull. By means of apparatus described in his book,[4] this physiologist was enabled to let the brain-pulse record itself directly by a tracing. The intra-cranial blood-pressure rose immediately whenever the subject was spoken to, or when he began to think actively, as in solving a problem in mental arithmetic. Mosso gives in his work a large number of reproductions of tracings which show the instantaneity of the change of blood-supply, whenever the mental activity was quickened by any cause whatever, intellectual or emotional. He relates of his female subject that one day whilst tracing her brain-pulse he observed a sudden rise with no apparent outer or inner cause. She however confessed to him afterwards that at that moment she had caught sight of a skull on top of a piece of furniture in the room, and that this had given her a slight emotion.

The fluctuations of the blood-supply to the brain were independent of respiratory changes,[5] and followed the quickening of mental activity almost immediately. We must suppose a very delicate adjustment whereby the circulation follows the needs of the cerebral activity. Blood very likely may rush to each region of the cortex according as it is most active, but of this we know nothing. I need hardly say that the activity of the nervous matter is the primary phenomenon, and the afflux of blood its secondary consequence. Many popular writers talk as if it were the other way about, and as if mental activity were due to the afflux of blood. But, as Professor H.N. Martin has well said, "that belief has no physiological foundation whatever; it is even directly opposed to all that we know of cell life."[6] A chronic pathological congestion may, it is true, have secondary consequences, but the primary congestions which we have been considering follow the activity of the brain-cells by an adaptive reflex vaso-motor mechanism doubtless as elaborate as that which harmonizes blood-supply with cell-action in any muscle or gland.

Of the changes in the cerebral circulation during sleep, I will speak in the chapter which treats of that subject. (James, 1890, pp. 97–99)

Note how carefully James considers the methodology and validity of Mosso's experiments, and with what restraint he interprets the results. Nonetheless, his conclusion is dramatic: "We must suppose a very delicate adjustment whereby the circulation follows the needs of the cerebral activity. Blood very likely may rush to each region of the cortex according as it is most active." This is a very modern insight indeed. By itself, it provides the basis to a contemporary observer for the claim that Mosso was the pioneer in establishing the new science of brain imaging.

It remains to note that Mosso went on to establish himself as one of the most prolific experimental physiologists of his time, contributing landmark studies summarized in a series of widely read books, which are summarized in Table 1.

As can be seen in Table 1, Mosso's interests, beginning with the physiology of the peripheral circulation and the physiology of the circulation of the brain, expanded to the physiological manifestations of emotional states, the temperature of the brain (a subject closely allied to blood flow), physiological adaptations to high altitude, books for the general public, and his final passion, the archeology and the prehistory of the Mediterranean people. All in all, he was one of the leading physiologists of his time, with a worldwide reputation.

Evidence for his international stature in science was the celebration of the decennial of the founding of Clark University in Massachusetts in 1899, highlighted by a symposium of leading scientists of the time (Story and Wilson, 1899). These included the physiologist Mosso along with the physicist Ludwig Boltzmann, founder of statistical mechanics; Santiago Ramon y Cajal, soon to receive the Nobel Prize in medicine; August Forel, an early pioneer of the neuron doctrine; and Henri Picard, a leading mathematician.

At the Clark celebration, the scientists gave public lectures on their main topics. Building on themes established in the present volume, Mosso chose to discuss "Psychic Processes and Muscular Exercise" and "The Mechanism of the Emotions." His interest in the first subject was motivated by his concern for improving children's education, as well as the conditions of workers. In the contemporary press coverage (Science, 12: 312, 1899) it was reported that

Table 1 SELECTED BOOKS AND MONOGRAPHS BY ANGELO MOSSO

1879 Die Diagnostik des Pulses (The Diagnosis of the Pulse)

1881 Der Kreislauf des Blutes im menschlichen Gehirn (Circulation of the Blood in the Human Brain, translated by C. N. Fabbri, ed. G. M. Shepherd, & M. E. Raichle)

1884 Sulla paura (Fear, translated by E. Lough & F. Kiesow, London, 1896)

1891 La fatica (Fatigue, translated by M. A. Drummond & W. B. Drummond, New York, 1904)

1894 La Temperatura del cervello (The Temperature of the Brain)

1897 Fisiologia dell' uomo sulle Alpi (Third edition, 1909) (Physiology of Man in the Alps)

1903 Mens Sana in Corpore Sano (Healthy Mind in Healthy Body)

1905 Vita moderna degli Italiani (Modern Life of Italians)

1907 Excursioni nel mediterraneo e gli scavi di Creta (Second edition, 1910) (English translation: The Palaces of Crete and their Builders, New York, 1908)

1910 La preistoria: le origini della civiltà mediterranea (The Dawn of Mediterranean Civilization, English translation by M. C. Harrison, New York, 1911)

. . . he sought to show how intimately related are mental processes and movements. . . . We might say that physical education and gymnastics serve not
only for the development of the muscles, but for that of the brain as well. . . .
No absolute local separation of movement and sensibility is demonstrable.

In the second talk, ". . . The seat of the emotions of joy and sorrow seems to
Professor Mosso to lie undoubtedly in the so-called sympathetic system." He
focuses especially on the bladder as an example of a vital organ that exhibits
"the most delicate reflex movements which occur in the organism." The bladder
contracted not only to very slight emotional stimuli but also to changes in the
organism instigated by problems of mental arithmetic.

Note that such a conclusion seems to parallel almost exactly the same sensitivity to "slight emotional stimuli" and mental exertions that he observed in the
circulation to the brain. This reflects the breadth of Mosso's approach to physiology, taking into account the whole organism in assessing physiological changes
underlying behavior.

Despite his enormous energy and many interests, his health began to fail
as he entered his 60s, and he had to give up his long-standing passion for
high-altitude studies. He turned instead with equal zeal to excavations of early
Mediterranean civilizations in southern Italy and Crete. These were summarized in his last book, published in the year of his death on November 24, 1910,
when he was 64.

NOTES

1. A. Mosso, Die Diagnostik des Pulses. Leipzig, 1879.
2. Francois-Franck, Fonctions Motrices, Leçon XXII.
3. La Paura (1884), p. 117.
4. Ueber den Kreislauf des Blutes im menschlichen Gehirn (1881). The Introduction
   gives the history of our previous knowledge of the subject.
5. In this conclusion M. Gley (Archives de Physiologie, 1881, p. 742) agrees with
   Professor Mosso. Gley found his pulse rise one to three beats, his carotid dilate, and
   his radial artery contract during hard mental work.
6. Address before Med. and Chirurg. Society of Maryland, 1879.

REFERENCES

Di Giulio C, Daniele F, Tipton C (2006) Angelo Mosso and muscular fatigue: 116 years
   after the first congress of physiologists: IUPS commemoration. Adv Physiol Educ
   30:51–57.
Haymaker W, Schiller F, eds (1970) The Founders of Neurology, One Hundred and
   Forty-Six Biographical Sketches by Eighty-Eight Authors. Springfield IL: Charles C
   Thomas.

Hoff H, Guillemin R (1967) Claude Bernard and the vasomotor system. In: Claude Bernard and Experimental Medicine (Grande F, Visscher M, eds), pp 75–104. Cambridge MA: Schenkman Publishing Company.

James W (1890) The Principles of Psychology. New York: Henry Holt & Company.

James, W. What is an emotion? Mind 9:188–205, 1884.

Shepherd G (1991) Foundations of the Neuron Doctrine. New York: Oxford University Press.

Story W, Wilson L, eds (1899) Clark University. 1889-1899. Decennial Celebration. Worcester MA: Clark University.

Zago S, Ferrucci R, Marceglia S, Priori A (2009) The Mosso method for recording brain pulsation: the forerunner of functional neuroimaging. Neuroimage 48:652–656.

COMMENTARY: FROM MOSSO TO MODERN BRAIN IMAGING

Some may wonder why a book on brain blood flow and its relationship to brain function in humans written over 130 years ago would be of interest now, given the sophistication of our present technology and experimental strategies in mapping the human brain. Our answer is twofold. First, we should not forget how the richness of the past has influenced the present. In this regard we repeat the words of Angelo Mosso who, in the introductory chapter of his book, graciously said, "I shall, whenever I think it advisable, tie certain critical considerations to the historical data, above all to highlight certain scientific accomplishments of our predecessors and to pluck from ill-deserved oblivion those which in physiology have prepared and paved the way for the view nowadays considered established" (p. 6—hereinafter the page numbers refer to the translated text). It is clear to us that with few exceptions, Mosso's accomplishments have suffered from ill-deserved oblivion. It is our hope that the translation of his book on brain circulation will serve to rectify that situation. In Figure 2 we provide a chronology of events leading from Mosso's original work to current brain activity mapping.

Our second motivation in preparing this translation was to make available a view of a truly remarkable scientist. As noted previously in the Brief Biography, Mosso was an internationally acclaimed scientist in his day, yet he is virtually unknown today. To understand how he achieved that stature, it is important to "see him in action" as a scientist. This book, translated for the first time into English, will allow you to see him in action and understand what it takes to do great, truly innovative science.

We note that Mosso subsequently explored human brain function by measuring local brain temperature changes (La Temperaturea del cervello [1894] Milano) and shifts in the distribution of body weight, which he attributed to the redistribution of blood flow from body to brain (Applicazione della bilancia allo studio della circolazione sanguigna dell' uomo [1894] Atti della R Acad Lincei Mem Cl Sci Fis Mat Nat XIX:531-543). However, the work contained in this translation of his text on brain pulsations and behavior best exemplifies his most relevant contributions to modern functional brain imaging and the field of cognitive neuroscience.

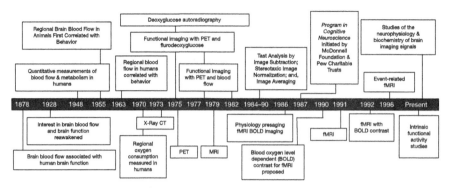

Figure 2 Timeline - Study of Cerebral Circulation

To begin, Mosso's general perspective regarding his studies of the blood circulation in the brain and of the "cerebral movements" it controls should be understood. Again, this is best captured in his own words (p. 107):

The fluctuations of the mental functions with decreasing or increasing blood flow to the brain form the subject of one of the most interesting studies, with which the psychologist is able to engage with experimentally: for there is no other way in which the intimate connection between the psychic and material functions of the organism can be more visibly evidenced. It is enough to diminish the blood supply to the brain by just a small amount, for consciousness to cease immediately. Should someone ask me, which among all organic functions were tied most closely to any even minimal change of the metabolism, I would answer without hesitation: consciousness.

Mosso continues:

The molecular equilibrium in the organs, which are the seat of reason, is deeply upset already by influences that in no perceptible way disturb the functions of other body parts, because tissue metabolism in the brain takes place more actively, and the makeup of constituent materials is more unstable. The higher value of psychic phenomena lies in the greater complexity of the events upon which they are based. One must also not be surprised if, as many others, I am inclined to consider the mind as the noblest expression of organic activity simply because of all the manifestations of the organism, it most appears as servant of the metabolic substance.[1] (p. 137)

We begin with Angelo Mosso's seminal observation in his laboratory in Turin on Monday morning, September 23, 1878. In the laboratory with Professor Mosso was 37-year-old Michele Bertino, "a peasant of sturdy build" who a year before had been struck on the head by a falling brick at a construction site. Although the wound to the scalp had healed completely, the injury had left Bertino with a rather large bony defect in the skull over the right prefrontal cortex. Mosso was interested in Bertino because Bertino's bony defect permitted recordings to be made of the pulsations of the brain, an opportunity Mosso leapt at because of his ongoing research on circulatory pulsations in other parts of the body, as was also being carried out by others in Europe. As was usual in the Mosso laboratory, Bertino was instrumented with unique devices of Mosso's design that permitted simultaneous and continuous recordings of brain pulsations (Figure 1—here and elsewhere these refer to the figure numbering in the original text) and, importantly, arterial pulsations in the forearm (Figure 2).

The recording session with Bertino was proceeding in the usual manner when the clock in the room struck 12 and at the same time one could hear the bell in the neighboring church. As Mosso noted, the unexpected impact of these sounds was a dramatic increase in the pulsations recorded from Bertino's brain. Mosso's reaction is best recorded in his own words (p. 52):

> Since I had been struck by the extraordinary increase of the cerebral pulsa-
> tion after the ringing of the church bells had begun, especially since at the
> same time the radial (artery) pulse had only undergone a relatively minimal
> modification, I asked Bertino. . . whether he was in the habit of reciting the
> Ave Maria at noon time. This question occurred to me because of my sus-
> picion that the important change in the cerebral circulation when the clock
> struck twelve was possibly related to the emotion which manifested itself in
> the man because at noontime he could not, as it is the custom of our rural
> people, make the sign of the cross or say a prayer. In fact, Bertino's answer
> to me was that he at times recites the Ave Maria.

This remarkable and unexpected observation was followed immediately by what must arguably be the first attempt to relate changes in cerebral blood flow to changes in normal brain function in the human brain. As noted in Figure 19, Mosso asked Bertino to multiply 8 by 22, causing, after a delay of several seconds, another increase in brain pulsations over the right prefrontal cortex that gradually returned toward baseline only to increase again when Bertino responded with the answer.

Several features of the changes observed in Bertino's brain during the performance of the task posed by Mosso coincide with modern observations being made daily in cognitive neuroscience laboratories worldwide with functional magnetic resonance imaging (fMRI). Typical of such responses is a delay in the brain's vasculature response of several seconds, which is clearly shown in Figure 19. This is usually followed by an increase in activity that is highest initially (the so-called onset transient: M. D. Fox et al., 2005), which is followed by a sustained elevation in activity that is terminated at the completion of the task by an additional further increase in activity (the so-called offset transient), all of which is seen, remarkably, in the tracing of brain pulsations obtained from Bertino (Figure 19). The organ specificity of these observations is critically underscored by the absence of any appreciable change in the systemic blood pressure as recorded simultaneously in the forearm of Bertino, a testimony to the meticulous detail Mosso applied to experimental design.[2]

Mosso's Difficulty With His "Institutional Review Board"

At this point we draw the reader's attention to an observation made by Mosso with which every medical scientist studying patients will sympathize.

> Here I must regretfully recall a circumstance that nearly rendered impossible the execution of most of the experiments communicated in this work. On the first day, I had been given permission by the hospital that Bertino be allowed to come to my laboratory, and thus, at that time, I conducted with him a series of observations [that] are certainly among the most beautiful. Since then, however, the same permission was refused to me even though the man was well and strolled around the garden all day long. I was therefore required to set up shop in a hospital room where I was continuously busy merely with putting together my devices or else with taking them apart. In such circumstances I could naturally not think about arranging everything with all of the comfort necessary for such delicate experiments, and thus I had to refrain from many an interesting observation that I had intended to make. It is surely lamentable that in the largest hospital of the city such as Turin, scientific studies find so little encouragement. In this matter, one was until recently, still in a deplorable state of dependence upon clerics and nuns, who are in command of the hospitals. (p. 134)

Mosso's impressive work on the brain and its circulation garnered the attention of no less a figure than William James. As noted previously in the Brief Biography, in his monumental two-volume text *Principles of Psychology* (James, 1890), James has an entire chapter "On Some General Conditions of Brain Activity" wherein he states, "All parts of the cortex, when electrically excited, produce alterations both of respiration and circulation" (Volume 1, p. 97). This remarkably foresighted statement for its time explicitly references the work of Mosso (for some additional details see endnote[3]).

Despite a promising beginning, interest in the relationship between brain function and brain blood flow virtually ceased during the first quarter of the 20th century. Undoubtedly, this was due in part to a lack of tools sufficiently sophisticated to pursue this line of research. In addition, the work of Leonard Hill, Hunterian professor of the Royal College of Surgeons in England, was probably influential (Hill, 1896). His eminence as a physiologist overshadowed the inadequacy of his own experiments that wrongly led him to conclude that no relationship existed between brain function and brain circulation.

There was no serious challenge to Leonard Hill's views until John Fulton reported a remarkable clinical study of a patient, Walter K., in the 1928 issue of the journal *Brain* (Fulton, 1928). During the course of his evaluation and treatment for a vascular malformation lying over his visual cortex, Walter K. remarked to his physicians that a noise (i.e., bruit) that he perceived in the back of his head increased in intensity when he was using his eyes. He said that he had often noticed this during the preceding several years but had "never thought much of it." As Fulton commented:

> It was not difficult to convince ourselves that when the patient suddenly began to use his eyes after a prolonged period of rest in a dark room, there was a prompt and noticeable increase in the intensity of his bruit. Activity of his other sense organs, moreover, had no effect upon his bruit. The conclusion drawn from this remarkable case was that blood flow to visual cortices was sensitive to the attention paid to objects in the environment.

It was not until the end of World War II that Seymour Kety and his colleagues opened the next chapter in studies of brain circulation and metabolism. In 1948, Kety and Carl Schmidt (1948) developed the first quantitative method for measuring human *whole* brain blood flow and metabolism. Their work provided the first quantitative measurement of the enormous burden the brain places on the energy budget of the body. They documented that while the brain is only 2% of the body weight, it consumes 20% of the energy. Interestingly, Mosso demonstrated the unique sensitivity of the brain to its nutritional requirements many years before.[4]

Because Kety and Schmidt's initial measurements were confined to the whole brain, they were not suitable for brain mapping. However, in 1955, Kety and colleagues introduced an in vivo tissue autoradiographic measurement of *regional* blood flow in laboratory animals (Landau et al., 1955), which provided the first glimpse of quantitative *regional* changes in blood flow in the brain related directly to brain function, just as Mosso had predicted. Derivatives of this tissue autoradiographic technique many years later became important for the measurement of blood flow in humans with positron emission tomography (PET), which provided a means of quantifying the spatial distribution of radiotracers in tissue without the need for invasive autoradiography (see later).

In 1963, following up on the important early observations by Kety and colleagues, a pair of Scandinavian investigators, David Ingvar (Sweden) and Niels Lassen (Denmark), and their colleagues collaboratively devised methods for the measurement of regional cerebral blood flow in humans (Ingvar and Risberg, 1965). That regional cerebral blood flow reflects the mental state of humans was clear from their work and that of others (for a review of this work see Lassen et al., 1978). In 1970, it became possible for the first time to relate regional oxygen consumption in the human brain to blood flow as well (Ter-Pogossian et al., 1970).

In 1973, X-ray computed tomography (X-ray CT) was introduced by its inventor Godfrey Hounsfield (1973). It is hard to overestimate the importance of this invention for clinical medicine, as well as being a critical stimulus for the development of other imaging technologies. In creating CT, Hounsfield had arrived at a practical solution to the problem of producing three-dimensional transaxial tomographic images of an intact object from data obtained by passing highly focused X-ray beams through the object and recording their attenuation. Hounsfield's invention received enormous attention and quite literally changed the way in which we looked at the human brain. Gone, also, were difficult-to-interpret, unpleasant, and sometimes dangerous clinical techniques like pneumoencephalography. CT was, however, an anatomical tool. Function was to be the province of PET and MRI.

The first out of the box in 1975 was positron emission tomography, or PET, which was developed (Phelps et al., 1975; Ter-Pogossian et al., 1975) to take advantage of the unique decay scheme of positron-emitting radionuclides (e.g., ^{15}O, ^{11}C, and ^{18}F). With PET, there was now a way to perform quantitative tissue autoradiography in humans obtaining detailed measurements of blood flow, metabolism, pharmacology, and biochemistry in health and disease (for review see Raichle, 1983).

Also in 1975, Louis Sokoloff and his colleagues at the National Institutes of Health introduced another activity marker in the form of 14C-2-deoxyglucose, which was to play a key role in studies of functional brain mapping in animals not possible in the human. This isotope of glucose, lacking an oxygen on the number 2 carbon atom, is taken up by cells and phosphorylated but is not a substrate for further metabolism in the cell. In large doses it had been used in experiments to block glucose metabolism. Sokoloff and colleagues labeled it with 14C and injected it into laboratory rats in tracer amounts. Because active cells for their energy needs are exquisitely dependent on glucose and oxygen delivered by the local vasculature, the labeled compound was trapped unmetabolized in the active cells and could be visualized by autoradiography to show locations where cells had been active. This technique provided our first detailed view of regional brain metabolism in the mammalian brain and its relationship to brain function.

The method was introduced by Kennedy et al. (1975; see also Sokoloff, 1984), who confirmed its validity by demonstrating, among other things, ocular dominance columns in monkey visual cortex. One of the first new findings with the method, reported in the same year, was evidence not seen before that in the awake rat, odor stimulation elicits activity patterns in the thin layer of glomeruli in the olfactory bulb (Sharp et al., 1975). Other new findings soon followed: mapping of focal seizures (Collins, 1978), circadian rhythms in the suprachiasmatic nucleus (Schwartz and Gainer, 1977), and changes in single barrels (Durham and Woolsey, 1977). The method could even be extended to invertebrates, demonstrating with tritiated deoxyglucose odor-elicited patterns in *Drosophila* (Rodrigues and Buchner, 1984) and labeling in single neurons in molluscs (Sejnowski et al., 1980). Animal experiments thus played a critical role in building the legacy of Mosso.

In 1979, the 14C-deoxyglucose technique was adapted for PET utilizing ^{18}F-fluorodeoxyglucose (Reivich et al., 1979; Phelps et al, 1979) and is now widely used in clinical medicine as well as in research. In 1982, the earlier-mentioned tissue autoradiographic technique for the measurement of regional brain blood flow in animals (Landau et al., 1955) was adapted to PET using $H_2^{15}O$, making up to 12 repeat measurements of brain function in a single setting (P. T. Fox et al., 1984) because of the short physical half-life of ^{15}O. The measurement time of blood flow was 1 minute, compared to 40 minutes for ^{18}F-fluorodeoxyglucose, greatly expanding the opportunity for brain activity mapping with PET.

From 1984 to 1990, there was an explosion of technical developments associated with functional brain mapping with PET, including task analysis by image subtraction, stereotaxic image registration and normalization, and image averaging (e.g., see Peterson et al., 1988). The development of these strategies became critical to the later development of fMRI.

In 1986, the first of two papers was published (P. T. Fox and Raichle, 1986; P. T. Fox et al., 1988) that surprised the brain blood flow and metabolism world by demonstrating with PET that when brain blood flow changes, it does so more than oxygen consumption. The result was that changes in brain activity were heralded by changes in the oxygenation of hemoglobin. Importantly, MRI is very sensitive to the oxygenation of hemoglobin (Pauling and Coryell, 1936), setting the stage for the later development of fMRI.

In 1990, Seiji Ogawa and his colleagues at Bell Laboratories proposed the use of deoxyhemoglobin as an MRI contrast agent for functional brain imaging and coined the term *BOLD* for blood oxygen level–dependent contrast. BOLD fMRI was, however, not the first functional imaging done with MRI. That occurred in 1991 when Jack Belliveau and his colleagues performed the first fMRI using an intravenously administered contrast agent (Belliveau et al., 1991). While this work signaled the arrival of fMRI, it could not compete with PET because only a limited number of measurements could be made in each subject due to the need to readminister the contrast agent. That all changed in 1992, when four groups almost simultaneously introduced BOLD fMRI (Bandettini et al., 1992; Frahm et al., 1992; Kwong et al., 1992; Ogawa et al., 1992).

From that time BOLD fMRI has transformed both animal and human studies of brain function. One driving force has been ever more powerful magnets, currently up to 7 Tesla for humans and 12 Tesla for animal experiments. This makes it possible to achieve resolutions far below the regional level, in the mouse down to 100-um voxels or below, enabling the investigation of changes in blood flow at the level of layers, barrels, and glomeruli (Yang et al, 1998; Xu et al., 2003). Use of two-photon microscopy in animal experiments is revealing blood flow changes in relation to sensory responses at the glomerular, cellular, and capillary level (Lecoq et al., 2009). At these levels, Mosso's early vision merges with modern cellular and molecular brain studies.

For cognitive studies in humans, the BOLD fMRI package was completed in 1996 with the introduction of event-related fMRI (Buckner et al., 1996), which freed investigators to employ the true sophistication of behavioral paradigms from cognitive psychology. The impact of fMRI on cognitive neuroscience has been remarkable. Since the introduction of fMRI, there have been nearly 13,000 refereed publications employing the technique largely but not exclusively in humans of all ages. Most of this work is being performed on MR instruments dedicated to research, in contrast to the early days in which work was done, after hours, on hospital instruments.

The study of human cognition with blood flow–based methods such as PET and MRI was aided greatly by the involvement of cognitive psychologists in the 1980s whose experimental designs for dissecting human behaviors using information-processing theory fit extremely well with emerging functional brain imaging strategies (Posner and Raichle, 1994). It may well have been the combination of cognitive psychology and systems neuroscience with brain imaging that lifted this work from a state of indifference and obscurity in the neuroscience community in the 1970s to its current role of prominence.

Remarkably, the basic behavioral strategy employed in this work was developed at almost the same time that Mosso was making his observations on the effects of behavior on brain circulation. This strategy for dissecting human behavior that became the centerpiece of functional brain imaging was based on a concept introduced by a contemporary of Mosso, the Dutch physiologist Franciscus C. Donders (for a recent review of his work in English, see Draaisma, 2002). In 1868, Donders proposed a general method to measure thought processes based on a simple logic. He subtracted the time needed to respond to a light (say, by pressing a key) from the time needed to respond to a particular color of light. He found that discriminating color required about 50 msec. In this way, Donders isolated and measured a mental process for the first time by subtracting a *control state* (i.e., responding to a light) from a *task state* (i.e., discriminating the color of the light). In the modern era of functional brain imaging, this strategy was first fully implemented in a study of single word processing (Petersen et al., 1988). Since then it has been exploited with exponentially increasing sophistication in the functional imaging world.

In 1987, a meeting attended by representatives of the scientific community and various research foundations was held at the headquarters of the James S. McDonnell Foundation in St Louis. At this meeting, it was decided that the time had come to explore the possibility of developing a new field of research that combined the quantitative measurement of behavior, as exemplified by the branch of psychology known as cognitive psychology, and systems neuroscience at the human level employing the rapidly developing techniques in functional brain imaging. After 2 years of planning, a program, largely focused on training, was initiated with funds from the McDonnell Foundation and the Pew Charitable Trusts. In addition to institutional and individual investigator funding, the program ran a summer workshop first at Harvard and then at Dartmouth. The McDonnell-Pew program in cognitive neuroscience continued for 13 years and quite literally created the field of cognitive neuroscience. A cadre of newly trained young people was prepared to take proper advantage of the developments in imaging and other cognitive methods.

Two important new directions have emerged.

First, one of the most remarkable discoveries to emerge from functional imaging of the brain is the role of ongoing or intrinsic activity. It consumes the vast majority of the brain's enormous energy budget (fully 20% of the body's energy requirements in adults) as compared to task-evoked activity (Raichle, 2010a, 2010b; Raichle and Mintun, 2006). Furthermore, this ongoing activity exhibits a remarkable degree of organization that can be interrogated through the spontaneous fluctuations in BOLD fMRI (M. D. Fox and Raichle, 2007; Raichle, 2010b, 2011) in subjects of all ages who are awake, asleep, or under general anesthesia. Its study also has revealed many new insights into the pathophysiology of disease (Zhang and Raichle, 2010). Mosso became aware of the importance of intrinsic activity during the course of the research reported in this book. Sleep formed the basis of his interest.

During Mosso's many research sessions, particularly with Bertino, he had occasion to observe periods of sleep. It should be recalled that our understanding of the neurophysiology of sleep did not begin until the first measurements of the human electroencephalogram (EEG) were performed by Hans Berger (1929) (for translations of his initial reports on the human EEG, see Gloor, 1969). The EEGs of sleeping subjects were noted early on to be dominated by slow, synchronous electrical activity, which was assumed to be the primary signature of sleep and, to this day, is referred to as slow-wave sleep (SWS). It was not until the work of Nathaniel Kleitman and his student Eugene Aserinsky (Aserinsky and Kleitman, 1953, reviewed in Shepherd, 2010) that rapid eye movement (REM) sleep became a recognized second component of normal sleep with its characteristic eye movements and awake-like EEG and its association with dreaming.

Remarkably, Mosso, working 50 to 75 years prior to the formal delineation of sleep stages, recognized two distinct phases of sleep as he recorded pulsations of the brain during sleep. Speaking of his observations during sleep, he noted that "... during sleep there is a period of such profound rest of the psychic centers that all conceptual activity, even the unconscious one,[5] comes to a complete halt. To such a period would correspond those portions of the pulse tracings in which the pulse contours become regular and uniform" (translation p. 72). It is very tempting to think that what Mosso refers to here is SWS. Significant reductions in brain circulation and metabolism have been clearly documented in SWS that are consistent with Mosso's observations (Boyle et al., 1994; Braun et al., 1997) along with regularization and slowing of the EEG.

In another passage (p. 66 in the translation), while he was recording from Bertino, Mosso makes the following observation (Bertino had been asleep, awoke briefly, and then fell back asleep while Mosso was making adjustments with his recording instruments): "A few seconds later I am able to resume recording and discover that the cerebral pulsations have reverted to their original configuration, the same as in the waking state at the start of the experiment." Obviously, this was a very different phase of sleep than that associated with pulse tracings that had become regular and uniform. It is very tempting to think that he recognized the earliest evidence of what we now call REM sleep, fully 75 years prior to its official recognition by Aserinsky and Kleitman.

Despite the several observations we have chosen to highlight and the many more that fill his book, it would have been impossible for Mosso and his contemporaries to imagine what their work foretold about brain activity mapping as we see it today. And the story continues to unfold. At present, the work includes not only the creation of brain maps during a countless variety of mental states including quiet repose and unconsciousness, in humans as well as in laboratory animals, but also how these maps change across the life span in health and disease. A critical challenge is to establish a deeper understanding of the nature of the brain imaging signals, particularly the BOLD signal, as a means of relating brain to behavior. This work includes attempts to understand not only its relationship to brain metabolism (Raichle and Mintun, 2006) but also its relationship to the underlying neurophysiology of individual neurons and microcircuits (e.g., see He et al., 2008; Logothetis et al., 2001). When thoughtfully considered, it has become apparent that all parties to this important endeavor need to pause and consider carefully how brain circulation, metabolism, biochemistry, and electricity relate to one another and to our understanding of human behavior. A call for such a broad-ranging view of science is not new or related just to the brain (e.g., see Smith, 1968).

In sum, as we harvest the fruits of our present labors and contemplate the future, we should have a deeper appreciation for the roles played by Mosso and the many other pioneers on whose shoulders we stand. We hope that the translation of this important early work will serve as a reminder of our debt to Angelo Mosso, an individual who truly exemplified what it means to be a great scientist. He was someone, to paraphrase his own words, whose accomplishments richly merit being plucked from undeserved neglect and made a model against which to judge our own advances.

NOTES

1. It is precisely this cue that Roy and Sherrington picked up on in their animal experiments, reported in 1890 in the *Journal of Physiology,* on factors influencing the brain circulation.
2. Ten years after the publication of Mosso's book, Roy and Sherrington published their often cited paper "On the Regulation of the Blood-Supply of the Brain." In that paper they acknowledge the work of Mosso but state that the primary weakness of his method was that he was unable to measure the pressure in the systemic arteries and veins! They obviously did not read carefully the details of his experiments wherein he points out that in order to interpret changes in the brain, it is important to monitor changes in other organs simultaneously along with changes in respiration, all of which he did with great care.
3. On page 98 of Volume 1 of the *Principles of Psychology,* James reproduces a tracing (Fig. 23) culled from Mosso's work. In this figure James labels tracing A as "during intellectual repose" and tracing B as "during intellectual activity." These tracings

are actually from Figure 12 in Mosso's book, of the right and left forearm! The correct figures would have been Figures 18 and 19 on pages 65 and 67, which detail the dramatic results of the experiment performed on Bertino as described previously and on pages XX through XX in the translated volume. This mistake has persisted through many reprintings of this famous work.

4. On page 142 of the translated text, Mosso notes: "The great sensitivity of the brain to any influences impairing nutrition is even more obviously manifest in our above mentioned experiment PET inasmuch as during it, 8 seconds were already enough for the blood supply. . . to reveal itself as inadequate for the preservation of the metabolic needs of the phenomenon of consciousness."

5. While pursuing his sleep studies, Mosso became fascinated by the unconscious processing of sensory information, noting that stimuli such as a touch or a sound that affected his measurements of brain pulsations did not awaken the subject. "The same changes that in the waking state are produced by mental activity in our body, also repeat themselves during sleep through external influences upon our sensory organs, even when such influences are unable to awaken us from sleep" (translation p. 70). "These alterations occurring without our knowledge constitute one of the most wonderful systems that we may be able to observe among the perfections of our organization. During the interruption of consciousness, our body is not helplessly exposed to the influences of the outside world, or left in danger of becoming prey to its enemies. Even during sleep, a part of the nervous centers monitors the influences of the external world and prepares in a timely manner the material conditions of our awakening" (translation p. 75).

REFERENCES

Aserinsky E, Kleitman N (1953) Regularly occurring periods of eye motility, and concomitant phenomena, during sleep. Science 118:273–274.

Bandettini PA, Wong EC, Hinks RS, Tikofsky RS, Hyde JS (1992) Time course EPI of human brain function during task activation. Magn Reson Med 25:390–397.

Belliveau JW, Kennedy DN Jr, McKinstry RC, Buchbinder BR, Weisskoff RM, Cohen MS, Vevea JM, Brady TJ, Rosen BR (1991) Functional mapping of the human visual cortex by magnetic resonance imaging. Science 254:716–719.

Berger H (1929) Über das Elektroenkephalogramm des Menschen. Arch Psychiat Nervenkr 87:527–570.

Boyle PJ, Scott JC, Krentz AJ, Nagy RJ, Comstock E, Hoffman C (1994) Diminished brain glucose metabolism is a significant determinant for falling rates of systemic glucose utilization during sleep in normal humans. J Clin Invest 93:529–535.

Braun AR, Balkin TJ, Wesenten NJ, Carson RE, Varga M, Baldwin P, Selbie S, Belenky G, Herscovitch P (1997) Regional cerebral blood flow throughout the sleep-wake cycle. An H2(15)O PET study. Brain 120 (Pt 7):1173–1197.

Buckner RL, Bandettini PA, O'Craven KM, Savoy RL, Petersen SE, Raichle ME, Rosen BR (1996) Detection of cortical activation during averaged single trials of a cognitive task using functional magnetic resonance imaging. Proc Natl Acad Sci U S A 93:14878–14883.

Collins RC (1978) Kindling of neuroanatomic pathways during recurrent focal penicillin seizures. Brain Res 150:503–517.

Draaisma D (2002) The Age of Precision: F.C. Donders and the Measurement of the Mind. Nijmegen, Netherlands: University of Nijmegen.

Durham D, Woolsey TA (1977) Barrels and columnar cortical organization: evidence from 2-deoxyglucose (2-DG) experiments. Brain Res 137:169–174.

Fox MD, Raichle ME (2007) Spontaneous fluctuations in brain activity observed with functional magnetic resonance imaging. Nat Rev Neurosci 8:700–711.

Fox MD, Snyder AZ, Barch DM, Gusnard DA, Raichle ME (2005) Transient BOLD responses at block transitions. Neuroimage 28:956–966.

Fox PT, Mintun MA, Raichle ME, Herscovitch P (1984) A noninvasive approach to quantitative functional brain mapping with H2 (15)O and positron emission tomography. J Cereb Blood Flow Metab 4:329–333.

Fox PT, Raichle ME (1986) Focal physiological uncoupling of cerebral blood flow and oxidative metabolism during somatosensory stimulation in human subjects. Proc Natl Acad Sci U S A 83:1140–1144.

Fox PT, Raichle ME, Mintun MA, Dence C (1988) Nonoxidative glucose consumption during focal physiologic neural activity. Science 241:462–464.

Frahm J, Bruhn H, Merboldt KD, Hanicke W (1992) Dynamic MR imaging of human brain oxygenation during rest and photic stimulation. J Magn Reson Imaging 2:501–505.

Fulton J (1928) Observations upon the vascularity of the human occipital lobe during visual activity. Brain 51:310–320.

Gloor P (1969) Hans Berger and the discovery of the electroencephalogram. Electroencephalogr Clin Neurophysiol Suppl 28:21–36.

He BJ, Snyder AZ, Zempel JM, Smyth MD, Raichle ME (2008) Electrophysiological correlates of the brain's intrinsic large-scale functional architecture. Proc Natl Acad Sci U S A 105:16039–16044.

Hill L (1896) The Physiology and Pathology of the Cerebral Circulation. An Experiment Research. London: J&A Churchill.

Hounsfield GN (1973) Computerized transverse axial scanning (tomography). 1. Description of system. Br J Radiol 46:1016–1022.

Ingvar DH, Risberg J (1965) Influence of mental activity upon regional cerebral blood flow in man. A preliminary study. Acta Neurol Scand Suppl 14:183–186.

James W (1890) The Principles of Psychology. New York: Henry Holt & Company.

Kennedy C, Des Rosiers MH, Jehle JW, Reivich M, Sharpe F, Sokoloff L (1975) Mapping of functional neural pathways by autoradiographic survey of local metabolic rate with (14C)deoxyglucose. Science 187:850–853.

Kety SS, Schmidt CF (1948) The nitrous oxide method for the quantitative determination of cerebral blood flow in man: theory, procedure and normal values. J Clin Invest 27:476–483.

Kwong KK, Belliveau JW, Chesler DA, Goldberg IE, Weisskoff RM, Poncelet BP, Kennedy DN, Hoppel BE, Cohen MS, Turner R, et al. (1992) Dynamic magnetic resonance imaging of human brain activity during primary sensory stimulation. Proc Natl Acad Sci U S A 89:5675–5679.

Landau WM, Freygang WH Jr, Roland LP, Sokoloff L, Kety SS (1955) The local circulation of the living brain; values in the unanesthetized and anesthetized cat. Trans Am Neurol Assoc 80:125–129.

Lassen NA, Ingvar DH, Skinhoj E (1978) Brain function and blood flow. Sci Am 239:62–71.

Lecoq J, Tiret P, Najac M, Shepherd GM, Greer CA, Charpak S (2009) Odor-evoked oxygen consumption by action potential and synaptic transmission in the olfactory bulb. J Neurosci 29:1424–1433.

Logothetis NK, Pauls J, Augath M, Trinath T, Oeltermann A (2001) Neurophysiological investigation of the basis of the fMRI signal. Nature 412:150–157.

Ogawa S, Tank DW, Menon R, Ellermann JM, Kim SG, Merkle H, Ugurbil K (1992) Intrinsic signal changes accompanying sensory stimulation: functional brain mapping with magnetic resonance imaging. Proc Natl Acad Sci U S A 89:5951–5955.

Petersen SE, Fox PT, Posner MI, Mintun M, Raichle ME (1988) Positron emission tomographic studies of the cortical anatomy of single-word processing. Nature 331:585–589.

Phelps ME, Hoffman EJ, Mullani NA, Ter-Pogossian MM (1975) Application of annihilation coincidence detection to transaxial reconstruction tomography. J Nucl Med 16:210–224.

Phelps ME, Huang SC, Hoffman EJ, Selin C, Sokoloff L, Kuhl DE (1979) Tomographic measurement of local cerebral glucose metabolic rate in humans with (F-18)2-fluoro-2-deoxy-D-glucose: validation of method. Ann Neurol 6:371–388.

Posner M, Raichle M (1994) Images of Mind. New York: W H Freeman and Company.

Raichle ME (2010a) The brain's dark energy. Sci Am 302:44–49.

Raichle ME (2010b) Two views of brain function. Trends Cogn Sci 14:180–190.

Raichle ME (2011) The restless brain. Brain Connect 1:3–12.

Raichle ME and Mintun MA (2006) Brain work and brain imaging. Annu Rev Neuroscience 29:449–476.

Reivich M, Kuhl D, Wolf A, Greenberg J, Phelps M, Ido T, Casella V, Fowler J, Hoffman E, Alavi A, Som P, Sokoloff, L (1979) The [18F]fluorodeoxyglucose method for the measurement of local cerebral glucose utilization in man. Circ Res 44:127–137.

Rodrigues V, Buchner E (1984) [3H]2-deoxyglucose mapping of odor-induced neuronal activity in the antennal lobes of Drosophila melanogaster. Brain Res 324:374–378.

Schwartz WJ, Gainer H (1977) Suprachiasmatic nucleus: use of 14C-labeled deoxyglucose uptake as a functional marker. Science 197:1089–1091.

Sejnowski TJ, Reingold SC, Kelley DB, Gelperin A (1980) Localization of[3H]-2-deoxyglucose in single molluscan neurones. Nature 287:449–451.

Sharp FR, Kauer JS, Shepherd GM (1975) Local sites of activity-related glucose metabolism in rat olfactory bulb during olfactory stimulation. Brain Res 98:596–600.

Shepherd G (2010) Creating Modern Neuroscience: The Revolutionary 1950s. New York: Oxford University Press.

Smith CS (1968) Matter versus materials: a historical view. Science 162:637–644.

Sokoloff L (1984) Metabolic Probes of Central Nervous System Activity in Experimental Animals and Man. Sunderland MA: Sinauer Associates.

Ter-Pogossian MM, Eichling JO, Davis DO, Welch MJ (1970) The measure in vivo of regional cerebral oxygen utilization by means of oxyhemoglobin labeled with radioactive oxygen-15. J Clin Invest 49:381–391.

Ter-Pogossian MM, Phelps ME, Hoffman EJ, Mullani NA (1975) A positron-emission transaxial tomograph for nuclear imaging (PETT). Radiology 114:89–98.

Xu F, Greer CA, Shepherd GM (2003) Odor maps in the olfactory bulb. J Comp Neurol 422:489–495.

Yang X, Renken R, Hyder F, Siddeek M, Greer CA, Shepherd GM, Shulman RG (1998) Dynamic mapping at the laminar level of odor-elicited responses in rat olfactory bulb by functional MRI. Proc Natl Acad Sci U S A 95:7715–7720.

Zhang D, Raichle ME (2010) Disease and the brain's dark energy. Nat Rev Neurol 6:15–28.

NOTES ON THE TRANSLATION

As has been noted before, German was the *lingua franca* for much of late 19th-century scientific research. The editors therefore chose to translate the 1881 German edition of Mosso's original *Sulla circolazione del sangue nel cervello dell'uomo; ricerche sfigmografiche* (1879, 1880). This edition closely followed the two original publications. In addition, careful comparison reveals that the German version amplifies some of Mosso's earlier material by providing further discussion and graphic illustration. It also includes a detailed introductory chapter on the history of the blood circulation in the brain.

The translation itself is essentially literal. Inasmuch as possible, the phraseology and style of the original manuscript are retained in an attempt to reflect most accurately the thought processes of the author. Chapter headings and subdivisions follow the original format. Details of footnotes and citations are reproduced in their entirety.

We have adjusted figure numbers to match corresponding chapters in order to improve readability. Also included in this English translation are a few translator's notes, to explicate terms or to provide added historical and cultural context for the modern reader.

Mosso's monograph conveys a detailed, day-by-day narrative of his investigations, affording the reader intimate opportunity to share in the author's experiments and findings just as they happened. Indeed, one gains a measure of insight into the creative scientific process, much in the way of the "investigative pathways" so painstakingly explored by my own early mentor in the history of science and medicine, the late Yale Professor Frederic L. Holmes.

I am much indebted to Dr. Gordon Shepherd for his close attention to many details of my translation, and for regular discussions of Mosso's experimental techniques and explorations. They contributed greatly to my understanding of the significance of this work. Moreover, Dr. Shepherd's unflagging enthusiasm for the project was infectious!

Translating one of the great works of 19th-century physiology has been both a privilege and a pleasure. It afforded me the opportunity to become acquainted with some of the life and work of an extraordinary man. Mosso was clearly a medical pioneer who committed himself to multifaceted inquiry for the whole of his working life. A prolific writer, he not only expanded his own scientific discipline but also brought his academic perspective to contemporary social issues of public health and hygiene, pedagogy and productivity, child labor, and the education of women.

For myself as translator and historian, Angelo Mosso was a fascinating figure. His death at the age of 64 was mourned by such luminaries as Ivan Pavlov, Charles Richet, and the poet Gabriele d'Annunzio. In 1908, two years before he died, Mosso had been nominated for the Nobel Prize in Physiology or Medicine for his "extensive work in physiology, especially studies of blood circulation, the bladder, temperature regulation of the brain, use of the plethysmograph and ergograph, and physiology of residents of the Alps." Mosso's ultimate premature demise may very well have forestalled this international recognition of his groundbreaking work.

Readers interested in further exploration of Mosso's life and career may wish to consult the Angelo Mosso Library at the University of Turin, fully digitized at http://vlp.mpiwg-berlin.mpg.de/references?id=lit25558.

Christiane Nockels Fabbri

BRIEF TRANSLATOR'S BIOGRAPHY

A native of Luxembourg, Christiane Nockels Fabbri completed her secondary education at the Lycée Hubert-Clément of Esch/Alzette. She studied psychology at Aix-en-Provence and medicine at Strasbourg. She was certified in Physician Associate Studies by the Yale School of Medicine and was awarded an MPhil in Medieval Studies and PhD in History of Medicine by Yale University. Her dissertation focused on medieval and early modern plague treatises. Dr. Nockels Fabbri currently practices at Yale Health in New Haven, CT, and is working on a history of medicine textbook.

Circulation of Blood in the Human Brain

INVESTIGATIONS BY A. MOSSO

PROFESSOR OF PHYSIOLOGY AT THE UNIVERSITY OF TURIN

WITH 87 TEXT ILLUSTRATIONS AND 9 TABLES

LEIPZIG

VEIT & COMP. PUBLISHERS

1881

IMPR. BY METZGER & WITTIG, LEIPZIG

To the Honorable Senator Jacob Moleschott.

Much beloved Professor,

Three years have already passed since I asked you for permission to dedicate this work to you. After you so kindly agreed, you will, I dare hope, forgive that I submit the same to you after such long delay.

No one knows better than you the sad events, which kept me for so long from this serious enterprise. First, I was afflicted by a grave illness, which would certainly have cost my life without your invaluable assistance and help. Later I sustained a much harder blow: I lost my dearly loved mother, on whose precious memory I may be permitted to call while I offer you this small token of my gratitude.

It pains me that I have not been able to produce a more accomplished work in order to show a worthier testimony of my appreciation to you who were my first teacher, and who knew to instill in me the thirst for knowledge and the love of learning.

Your devoted student
A. Mosso
Chieri, October 1880

TABLE OF CONTENTS

CRITICAL HISTORICAL INTRODUCTION

1

Although there is no shortage of valuable texts detailing in ample measure the literature on our subject (in which regard, among the most recent I must make particular mention of Althann's[1] and Salathé's[2] noteworthy treatises), and even though I myself had occasion, in a previous work,[3] to delineate the main features of the historical development of the question that will occupy us here, I nevertheless deem it necessary at this juncture, and for the purpose of comprehension, to preface the objective treatment of the cerebral blood circulation with a brief historical sketch. At the same time I shall, whenever I think it advisable, tie certain critical considerations to the historical data, above all to highlight specific scientific accomplishments of our predecessors and to pluck from ill-deserved oblivion those that in physiology have prepared and paved the way for the view nowadays considered as established: the view according to which the movements that are observed in the brain are in no way particular to the brain, but represent a phenomenon common to all organs and parts of the body and dependent on the circulation of the blood.

The history of our knowledge of the blood circulation in the brain and of the cerebral movements it controls can be summarily divided into three very uneven periods, of which the first begins in Greco-Roman antiquity and ends in the first half of the 18th century; the second, introduced by the studies of Schlichting (1750), concludes with Ravina in the first years of our century; and the third, which begins with Magendie (1825), has, in later years, with the utilization of more accurate measuring instruments and especially of the graphic method, entered a second phase. However, in the interest of factual argument, I shall not be able in my account to adhere exactly to the chronologic sequence, and thus the subdivisions of this chapter do not conform as much to the indicated time periods as to the critical requirements.

Plinius[4] reported that the brain of Zoroaster at his birth exhibited such strong pulsations that it was able to lift the hand resting upon it: "... eidem cerebrum ita palpitasse, ut impositam repelleret manum, futurae praesagio sapientiae"

[Trans.: "his very brain pulsated so much that it thrust back the imposed hand, a presaging of future wisdom."][5]

Galen,[6] in his books on the olfactory organ, spoke of the movements of the brain, on the function of the human body parts, and on the function of respiration, and he did not leave any doubt that he must have conducted appropriate experiments on this subject.

Oribasius, who lived approximately two centuries after Galen, described the movements of the brain in a chapter on the olfactory organ. He indicated that the brain contracts during inspiration and then explicitly added the following:[7]

> . . . which movement is visible in the newborn as well as in persons with gaps in their skull. The movement itself is thus natural and uninterrupted. However, there supervenes yet another [movement], which is clearly apparent in all animals: indeed, if one removes the bones of the skull, one discerns, so long as the animals are silent, a pulsating motion which follows the same rhythm as that of the arteries and of the heart; yet when they cry, the entire brain rises and swells up.

Since Oribasius was merely a capable compiler of medical works who copied Aristoteles, Rufus, and, in the cited passage—as Daremberg[8] remarks—Galen, we may assume that with those words he summarized the collective teachings on the movements of the brain according to the point of view of ancient physiology.

It is generally known that after the death of Galen, the development of science underwent a thousand-year-long hiatus during which, throughout the entire Middle Ages, Galen's name dominated medical practice and theory.

It was only in the 16th century that new experiments were conducted, albeit with little success. Thus, Fallopius[9] was less fortunate than Galen, whose authority he dared rebel against in writing that "such a movement is hindered by the entire brain substance and I myself, in spite of every effort and diligence, could not discern in the brain any pulsation."

Vesalius stated in a letter to Fallopius that he could not convince himself that the brain, as Galen had supposed, contracted and expanded within the cranial cavity according to the manner of the heart. While he could not totally deny all movement since he had in fact observed, during his numerous vivisections as well as in head injuries and on the fontanels of children, the rising and falling of the cranial contents and indeed beneath the dura mater, he ascribed these movements to the vessels branching within the pia mater and explicitly emphasized that the rich vascularity of the membrane encasing the cerebral hemispheres could impart to the brain "the pulsations, the appearance, and the nature of the arteries."[10]

After Vesalius, it was only in the year 1750 that a second period of accurate experiments and assiduous observations began. Schlichting,[11] a Dutch anatomist dissatisfied (as he himself said) with what he found in older and newer works, wanted to engage in experiments in order to search earnestly for the truth. Even though his experiments only confirmed the findings of Oribasius, they nevertheless had the great merit to have ushered in a new era in the experimental physiology of the movements of the brain. During his numerous vivisections conducted with many animal species, he always found that the brain hemispheres followed the rhythm of the respiratory movements: "Quoties expicatus sum sedulus, detracta superiore cranii parte, viventium cerebra, toties animadverti perspicue, in omni expiratione cerebrum universum ascendere, id est, intumescere, atque in quavis inspiratione illud descendere, id est detumescere." [Trans.: "As often as I painstakingly stripped off the superior portion of the skull from the living brain, each time I clearly observed that in every expiration the entire brain rises, that is, it swells up, and in each inspiration it sinks, that is, it becomes less swollen."]

Schlichting was vague regarding the cerebral movements corresponding to arterial pulsations, and he was unable to decide whether it was the air or the blood flowing in greater quantity to the brain that caused the brain to swell.

He emphasized that the brain did not completely fill the cranial cavity, a fact also known, by the way, to Galen, who had demonstrated that there exists between the dura mater and the cerebral surface an empty space in which the movements of the brain take place. Schlichting observed during his experiments that when consciousness was lost and respiration stopped, the movements of the brain also ended and the brain shrank to the point that a probe could be introduced between the meninges; as soon as respiration was restored, the hemispheres swelled up and their movements returned.

During the last century, the traditional belief (according to Lorry, first expressed by Rufus in Ephesus) prevailed in medicine that the movements observed in the brain pertain to the dura mater. Pacchioni[12] maintained that the dura mater was a muscle *sui generis, triventer et quadritendineus* [Trans.: with three bellies and four tendons]. Baglivi,[13] who similarly conducted multiple vivisections in order to research cerebral movements, not only completely subscribed to Pacchioni's views but also undertook the daring task, in his words, to determine whether the motion of the heart, since it is under the influence of the brain, might not itself depend on the systole and diastole of the dura mater. These errors were so successfully countered by Schlichting that they have completely disappeared from science.

Soon thereafter, Lamure, Haller, and Lorry undertook, by means of numerous and precise experiments, to investigate the causes of the cerebral movements. Lamure derived the rising of the brain from an expiratory congestion of venous blood in the jugular and vertebral veins, and to support his theory showed that the same phenomena can also be induced in a dead animal if one alternately exerts pressure on the ribs, then releases it.[14]

Albrecht Von Haller, in his *Physiology*, discussed, with the depth and erudition by which he surpassed all his contemporaries, the history of the science of cerebral movements; since we must restrict ourselves to a cursory mention of the most important relevant studies, we refer to his great work[15] those who wish to acquaint themselves more closely with the older literature of the topic. Haller's own experiments on the movements of the brain are recorded in his two famous treatises "On the Sensitive and Excitable Nature of the Body Parts of Animals," which he read to the Academy of Göttingen in 1752 and 1755. Therein he described the movements of the brain, which correspond to the contractions of the heart, and illuminated with astonishing depth and expertise the relationships between respiration, cardiac activity, pulmonary circulation, and the circulation of the blood within the central organs of the nervous system. We want to cite from these treatises a passage in which his conceptions of the mechanism of the cerebral movements are developed with the greatest clarity:[16]

> The phenomenon observed by Schlichting is by no means unique to the brain; it is merely dependent on the ease with which the blood during inspiration penetrates from the right chamber of the heart into the lung, and from the thus facilitated emptying of the great nerve trunks into the said heart chamber. During expiration on the other hand, the compressed lung cannot receive the blood; the large veins therefore cannot empty, they swell up, and this swelling extends itself to the brain which becomes overfilled with blood because it cannot rid itself of the same via the jugular veins.

Lamure and Haller had thus attributed the movements of the brain to the expiratory congestion of the venous blood in the brain, and to the draining of the blood facilitated during inspiration. Lorry was the first who also considered the influence that the cardiac impulse and consequently the influx of arterial blood accelerated by systole must exert on the cerebral mass. The clarity with which he knew how to sum up into a coherent whole an entire series of factors involved in bringing about these movements leads us to cite from his treatise the following passage *in extenso*. These words, which he wrote down a century ago, gain all the more weight since they also represent the contemporary scientific standpoint, and we are unable to add anything better. In his analytic discussion of the influence of respiratory movements and cardiac contractions on the brain, he states:[17]

> Nous avons observé deux mouvements dans le cerveau: l'un répond à celui du coeur, l'autre à celui de la respiration; les mouvements du coeur et de la respiration sont donc les agens qui le produisent. Voyons les effets mécaniques de ces mouvements sur le cerveau. [Trans.: We have observed two movements in the brain: one responds to that of the heart, the other to that of the respiration; the movements of the heart and of the respiration are thus the agents that produce them. Let us consider the mechanical effects of these movements on the brain.]
>
> Les artères sont toujours pleines de sang: on ne saurait donc augmenter la quantité de ce fluide dans ces vaisseaux, sans rendre leur diamètre plus considérable. Quand le coeur se contracte, il pousse le sang dans les artères, ce liquide agit avec plus de force sur leurs parois, et produit en elles une dilatation: cette dilatation est générale, et se fait remarquer au moment de la contraction du coeur jusque dans les moindres artères. . . .

[The arteries are always filled with blood: therefore, one could not increase the quantity of this fluid within these vessels without making their diameter more considerable. When the heart contracts, it pushes the blood into the arteries; this liquid acts with greater force on their walls and produces in them a dilatation: this dilatation is general, and is noticeable at the moment of the cardiac contraction up to the smallest arteries. The capacity of all the arterial distributions disseminated in one part and taken together thus becomes more considerable. During the dilatation of the heart, the fibers of the arteries, which had been brought to a certain point of distension, retract through their elasticity: in one word, the formerly dilated arteries contract and in part sustain the movement that the heart had imparted to the blood; thus, the capacity of all the disseminated arteries taken together diminishes during the dilatation of the heart, while it had augmented during the contraction of this muscle.

In the course of the cardiac contraction, the dilating force of the arteries tends to inflate and to distend, so to speak, all the organs to which the blood is carried, and even more so those which because of their softness and flexibility are less able to resist the force of the cardiac impulse.]

While Haller, Lamure, and Lorry went about their investigations, Domenico Cotugno in 1764 published his own work concerning the cerebrospinal fluid. We are citing here some remarks from his work *De ischiade nervosa*,[18] to which we will return again later, when we discuss the role of the cerebrospinal fluid in relationship to the brain movements.

Quidquid autem spatii est inter vaginam durae matris, et medullam spinalem, id omne plenum etiam semper est: non nube vaporosa; sed aqua, ei quidem simili, quam circa cor continet pericardium, quae caveas cerebri ventriculorum adimplet, quae auris labyrinthum, quae reliqua tandem complet corporis cava.

Nec tantum haec aqua complens ab occipite ad usque imum os sacrum tubum durae matris, quo spinalis medulla vaginatur, indique medullam ipsam constanter incingit; sed et in ipso redundat calvariae cavo, omniaque complet intervalla, que inter cerebrum, et durae matris ambitum inveniuntur.

[Trans.: What space there is between the sheath of the dura mater and the spinal medulla is always completely filled: not by vaporous air, but by water similar to that which the pericardium contains around the heart; that which fills the ventricular cavities of the brain, the labyrinths of the ear; and finally, that which fills the rest of the body cavity.

This water not only fills the tube of the dura mater from the occiput down to the sacral bone where it sheaths the spinal cord, constantly encircling the medulla itself, but also flows into the very cranial cavity and fills all spaces found between the brain and the expanse of the dura mater.]

Cotugno further emphasized that together with the shrinking of the brain mass, which takes place in certain disease states as well as, especially, in old age, the quantity of the water surrounding the brain increases, and he provides forthwith the necessary instructions for the observation and collection of this liquid.

He demonstrated its identity in the cranial cavity and in the vertebral canal, as well as its free transition from one cavity into the other, and he showed that it can be easily collected from a cadaver if one places the cadaver in a vertical position and opens the vertebral column near the loin.

In the course of repeating his experiments on approximately 20 cadavers to determine the quantity of cerebrospinal fluid, he noticed that this fluid flowed as well, in the case of an intact skull, from an opening made in the area of the loin: "Quod si, capite integro, lumborum vertebrae aperiantur, inclususque tubus durae matris incidatur, humor affatim emerget: ac postquam tanta humoris copia emersit, quanta ad locum incisum sponte descendit, si caput cadaveris attolatur quatiaturque, versus locum apertum, quasi nova scaturagine reserata, vis aquae uberior denuo redundabit." [Trans.: "But if, with the head left intact, the lumbar vertebrae are opened, and the inside sheath of the dura mater is incised, humor emerges in abundance: and after such amount of humor has emerged as will flow to the incised area, if then the head of the cadaver is raised up and shaken toward the opened spot, the stream of water will flow more forcefully as if through a new incision."][19]

This observation, which neither he himself nor anyone after him knew how to make use of, is important enough to merit our full attention. The fact that the cerebrospinal fluid flows out of an opening of the lumbar spine in the face of an intact skull, and even more importantly, that the outflow restarts anew if one lifts and shakes the head of the corpse, constitutes for us the most compelling proof for the fact that, within certain parameters, the volume of the brain can easily change, and that the movements that can be observed on an opened skull are similarly unobstructed in the case of a closed cranium.

We do not wish to dwell further upon the experiments Portal[20] conducted in France and that he described in a report to the Paris Academy of Sciences without bringing to light anything new with regard to the movements that concern us, except that the spinal medulla swells during expiration. Instead, we will immediately turn to the experiments published in 1799 by Richerand. This researcher distinguished within the brain two different movements: one that displaces and lifts the cerebral mass, while the other produces a generalized swelling and turgor of the same. The lifting movement depends, according to Richerand, on the diastole of the arteries coursing at the base of the skull, which with each pulsation drive the superimposed mass of the hemispheres upward; the second movement, on the other hand, is presumably controlled by respiration and by the subsequent stagnation of venous blood.[21] Even though earlier Senac[22] and others articulated a similar view regarding the mechanism of the cerebral movements, nevertheless, since Richerand this hypothesis did not go further than a theory merely based on anatomical considerations. Neither Bichat nor Burdach[23] nor others, who later followed this interpretation, could corroborate it with decisive experiments. According to their ideas, the movement of the brain synchronous with the contractions of the heart is rooted not in a swelling of the entire mass of the hemispheres, but rather in a quasi-passive elevation produced by the diastole of the underlying arteries. This concept rested on the experience that after the opening of the skull and the ligation of the vertebral arteries, the brain is lifted up each time one directs against it a jet of water through a syringe introduced into the carotid artery. It is entirely clear that such an experiment completely misses its purpose, for it does not at all exclude the filling and dilatation of the arteries that penetrate into the brain mass, and can thus in no way demonstrate that the rising of the brain is based exclusively or even mostly on the expansion of the arteries ending at the base of the skull. I found in my own experiments that in man, such movements are also produced when the head, through flexion of the neck and body, is inclined so far forward that the brain no longer weighs on the great arteries of the cranial base, as is postulated by the aforementioned theory. Moreover, the consistency of the cerebral matter is not such that it could propagate the pulsation of the underlying arteries. In order to bolster his theory, Richerand did not hesitate to discredit the experiments of Lamure, and also claimed that it was not Haller himself who conducted the experiments mentioned in his discussion of the role of respiration.[24]

Lamure, Haller, and Lorry had conducted their investigations nearly simultaneously, and in the course of a decade, from 1750 to 1760, the study of the movements of the brain quickly made the advances discussed previously. After a determination of the mechanism of the events and a clear description of the basic questions, the topic appeared to be more or less exhausted, and nearly half a century went by for science to make a new advance in this field. It was an Italian, Dr. Antonio Ravina (born in the small village of Gottasecca, in the district of Mondovì in Piedmont, where he was a medical practitioner), who first attempted by means of new experiments to arrive at a closer evaluation of the conclusions reached by his predecessors. In his treatise *Specimen de motu cerebri*, published in February of 1811 in the Acts of the Academy of Sciences of Turin, we encounter the description of many astute observations and ingenious experimental methods, a number of which, having been forgotten, had to be invented a second time by later physiologists.

Among others, I want to mention a series of experiments by which Ravina sought to determine whether the movements of the brain would continue if, after opening the skull, the breach was covered with a glass plate and the contents of the skull thus withdrawn from the atmospheric pressure. These experiments are for us all the more interesting, for through them the merit accrues to our compatriot to have been first to conceive an idea that was to be taken up again much later by one of the most outstanding physiologists of modern times, Prof. Donders. Ravina, by means of a trephine, drilled into the skull an opening wide enough to introduce a wooden hollow cylinder, which he fastened and sealed from the air with cement made of oil, wax, and turpentine. The cylinder was equipped with a screw-on cover removable at discretion. In attaching a watch glass to the top of the cylinder and ensuring that this would hermetically seal the cranial cavity, Ravina nevertheless was able to observe the movements of the brain take place as before:

> Utebar alias vitro exiguo horologii, cum memorato cylindro superius aprime connexo, et tunc oculis intueri etiam licuit cerebrum turgescere in expiratione animantis, detumescere dein in inspirationis stadio, deprimi, et inferius revera descendere. Intra cavum cylindri aerem non admitti certior eram factus; cum etenim valide insufflarem per ferream exiguam fistulam, cylindro rite connexam, et sub experimentis affabre clausam, nullibi animadvertere potui aërem egredi, nec circa cylindri cum capite commissuram, nec alibi.
>
> [Trans.: At another time I used a small watch glass connected to the top of the aforementioned cylinder, and I was then able to observe with my own eyes the brain of the living creature swell in expiration, thereupon contract in the stage of inspiration, pressed down, and in reality descend inferiorly. I had made certain that no air entered the hollow of the cylinder, for indeed, even though I would blow forcefully through a small iron pipe duly connected to the cylinder, nowhere, up to the end of the experiment, could I notice any air escape, not near the juncture of the cylinder with the head nor anywhere else.][25]

Naturally there remained between the glass and the brain an airspace, which defeated the purpose of the experiment.

In order to solve some questions about the amplitude of the brain movements, Ravina used an apparatus, which I will describe later, and with which he could very accurately read, by means of a graduated gauge, by how much the brain volume increased or decreased during the respiratory movements. Not content with this stratagem, he chose another, equally ingenious method, which later on was likewise to be heralded as an invention of other physiologists; not only was Ravina's name forgotten, but also that of Lorry, who to my knowledge was the first to fit an artificially created cranial breach with an airtight glass tube, therein to pour liquid, the level of which would then rise and fall with the lifting and lowering of the brain. This is how Ravina proceeded:

> Majori, quam fieri potuerit, diligentia perforavi cranium canis maximae molis quidem, sed junioris adhuc aetatis. Quod abscidi rotundissimum osseum ex cranio circulum, rotundo foramine terebravi; atque huic foramini tubum vitreum diametri lineae unius ferruminavi, in parvum infundibulum superius desinentem. Dura meninge circa vulneris oram summa manu diligentissime resecta, ne superstes divelletur ab adhaesionibus suis, circulum osseum denuo adaptavi propria in sede, ibique firmissimis ligamentis retinebatur. Dein tubum vitreum aqua replebam. Facta tunc animanti facultate, ut duceret animam, aqua omnis ex tubo evanuit, et super cerebrum

se se diffudit sub inspiratione: at, dum expiravit animal, in tubo iterum apparuit aqua sanguine tincta, ut sub inspiratione iterum evanesceret.

[Trans.: With the greatest possible care I perforated the skull of a dog of considerable size, but still of young age. Insofar as I had removed a perfectly round circle of bone from the skull, I had bored through it a round aperture; to this I cemented a glass tube of a one-line diameter, which at the top ended in a small funnel. Having carefully resected the hard meninges around the wound orifice so that the remainder would not be torn from its attachments, I adjusted the bony circle once more in its proper place, where it had been held fast by extremely firm ligaments. Next I filled the glass tube with water. Having thus created the means in the live creature to draw breath, all the water would disappear from the tube, and disperse over the brain during inspiration: but when the animal exhaled, water tinged with blood appeared again in the tube, while during inspiration it once more vanished.][26]

Equally important are the experiments Ravina performed to demonstrate the changes of the brain movements depending on the position of the body. If, following trepanation of the skull, an animal was hung by its hind legs, the movements of the brain were made impossible to differentiate by the specific gravity (*Eigenschwere*) of the blood and by the obstructed venous outflow, whereas they were most clearly pronounced when the animal retained its usual posture. The variable intensity of these movements in different animal species depends, according to Ravina, on the unequal number of cerebral convolutions and on the commensurately different vascularity of the cerebrum.

With Ravina concludes the second period in the history of our subject. During the entire third period, which stretches to our time, the lack of new investigative methods posed a great obstacle to the rapid development of this branch of physiology.

2

Soon after the death of Bichat, Magendie emerged, whose influence in the field of experimental medicine was to hold sway for many years. While we recognize his eminent merit in singlehandedly toppling the vitalist ideas of the school of Bichat, we must nevertheless admit that his writings on the cerebrospinal fluid are the least accomplished of his works.[27] In his lectures held at the Institut de France in 1825 and 1826, and in the volume he himself collected of his lectures on this topic later on (1842),[28] he speaks of the cerebrospinal fluid as his own discovery and does not hesitate, in spite of Cotugno's research, to designate the aforementioned fluid as "a newly recognized element of our organism." His dislike of historic-literary investigations, to which he somewhat cavalierly admitted on this occasion, hardly excuses this disregard for foreign achievements.[29]

Jodin[30] attempted in vain to cover up the grave plagiarism of his teacher by compromising himself with a rather unfaithful translation of some important passages from Cotugno's work *De ischiade nervosa*. However, while one may argue that Magendie did not enrich the physiology of cerebral movements with any momentous facts, it is not to be underestimated that his studies substantially advanced the anatomical knowledge of the serous membranes of the central organs of the nervous system. He already emphasized that local changes in the cerebrospinal fluid on the brain surface would be very limited and showed that in man, depending on the time elapsed between death and autopsy, a significantly different quantity of this fluid is found.

Furthermore, it is to him that we owe the proof that this fluid is within the subarachnoid spaces at the surface of the brain and the spinal medulla, and these spaces he investigated and described in such detail that these studies alone would have sufficed to secure him one of the foremost places among anatomists.

The occurrence of cerebral movements in the intact skull had already been hypothesized by Galen, later by Schlichting[31] and Lamure,[32] and deemed possible at least in individual cases by Lorry,[33] because with its increase in volume the brain can expel blood from the surrounding veins. Haller did not completely deny these movements, and Ravina first specifically sought to demonstrate these movements in the intact skull, the brain being thus withdrawn from the pressure of the atmospheric air, which later Burdach, Magendie, Flourens, Ecker, and others also acknowledged in the presence of an intact skull. The occurrence of these movements, however, was declared impossible by other, no less capable, researchers.

For the sake of succinctness, we forego tracing the origin of this latter belief and begin our critical considerations with the next stage, when some were attempting to provide this very notion with the semblance of an experimental foundation. Fabre,[34] Monro,[35] Abercrombie,[36] Kellie,[37] and other authors of the Edinburgh School believed that, based on theoretical considerations, the skull contained always the same amount of blood and that a variation in volume of the central organs of the nervous system was utterly impossible.

The question of the brain movements, which, as we will see, will become all the more intricate and difficult the more we delve into the tangle of its factors and causative moments, was for them a very simple physical problem whose solution posed no difficulty, for in their view the skull represented a firm and rigid box, filled with an incompressible content (blood and brain matter).

Bergmann,[38] in accordance with this theory, tried to explain the blood circulation in the brain by comparing the cranium to an inflexible, water-filled box wherein the vascular system is represented by an elastic tube that enters through an opening of the box, runs through the entire cavity, and exits through another opening, but that is, however, hermetically fastened to the rim of both apertures so that the watery content of the box cannot come into direct contact with the atmospheric air. With this schema, he thought to provide evidence that in the intact skull, while blood circulates briskly through the elastic tubes (cerebral vessels), any amount of pressure could be imparted to this fluid and to the surrounding mass of the central nervous system organs without increase or decrease in the amount of blood contained in the vessels.

The diminished resistance of the vessels could not lead to any significant dilatation but could only engender increased pressure on the mass of the brain, and thus any increase of the blood volume would be impossible unless the cerebrospinal fluid had previously been reduced by a corresponding amount.

It is not surprising that such a simple argument, which by all appearances rested on indisputable physical considerations, was greeted by the medical community with enthusiasm and was used for the foundation of a new theory of cerebral diseases, along with a total refashioning of the concept of cerebral congestion.

To give an example of the exaggerations to which this theory led, I shall only mention that Hamernik[39] had no misgivings about comparing the vascular system of the brain with the metallic pipes of drinking water. According to his representations, the circulation in the bony skull took place according to the principle of a composite lever and was initiated by thoracic aspiration, while cardiac activity was completely negligible and positive arterial pressure was not present at all.

Abercrombie[40] taught that there are circulatory disturbances of the brain that are necessarily tied to compression of the hemisphere, since the arteries, when they expand under the pressure of the blood, compress the veins and hinder venous outflow, which must have as a consequence an increase in intracranial pressure. Not only was it believed that the brain was not subject to atmospheric pressure, but also there were even those who asserted that an animal, which is allowed to exsanguinate, dies of cerebral stroke.

3

In order to demonstrate that the brain, also in its normal state (i.e., with intact bony skull), at a minimum effects slower movements consisting of changes in its volume, it is sufficient to bring to mind some experiments that prove that even in a closed cranium the blood contained within the brain mass and its envelopes is subjected to very significant fluctuations. Burow[41] took two rabbits, killed them with cyanide, and, before cardiac contractions had stopped, strung up one by its ears and the other by its hind legs. After 24 hours he went about opening the skull of both animals: in the rabbit that had been hung up by its ears, brain and meninges were found to be pale, and sinuses and other cerebral vessels were empty; in the other, the brain was markedly hyperemic, dark red, with expanded cerebral sinuses, and with replete cerebral and meningeal vasculature.

Kussmaul and Tenner[42] compared the condition of the brain of two animals killed simultaneously, one by exsanguination, the other by strangulation after prior transsection of the cervical portion of the sympathetic trunk. The authors maintained that they had never seen such intense congestion of the brain matter and of the meninges as in the latter animal. So as not to deny value to these investigations perhaps for the sole reason that they were conducted after the death of the animal, we want to cite one more experiment, namely, that described by Th. Ackermann in his *Investigations of the Influence of Asphyxiation on the Quantity of Blood in the Brain and in the Lungs.*[43]

Here the process involved was similar to that used in Ravina's experiments, where the surface of the brain was observed through a window fashioned in the wall of the skull and hermetically closed with a glass. If the trachea was compressed, Ackermann saw the pink color of the brain become gradually bluish and cyanotic, while at the same time the diameter of the more significant vessels increased visibly; however, after respiration was restored, the brain regained its pale rose color and the vessels constricted again. If shutting of the trachea was continued, one would see, approximately 10 to 20 seconds before death, the cyanotic discoloration of the brain become increasingly pale and the ischemia of the brain attain its maximum within the first hour after strangulation, when the large vessels contracted to half their diameter.

Since we are certain that the vascular content of the brain can fluctuate significantly even in the intact skull, it is of interest for us to see how one has sought to explain this fact.

Above all, the most important condition was understood to lie in the local changes of the cerebrospinal fluid, namely, in the flowing of the latter out of the cranial cavity into the spinal canal and back.

Meanwhile, Magendie had already emphasized, as we saw earlier, that these displacements of the cerebrospinal fluid are very limited; and from my own experiments with human subjects I believe that I may draw the same conclusion; indeed, I believe for these and for other important reasons that the local variations of the said liquid are, under physiologic circumstances, of much lesser consequence for the conditions of the cerebral circulation than is generally assumed by physiologists even nowadays. In the course of my numerous observations of the blood circulation in the brain, and given normal nutrition of this organ, I did not encounter a single phenomenon that I thought I could attribute to a local alteration of the cerebrospinal fluid in the cranial cavity. I hope that my experiences regarding the pulse of the blood coming out of the cranial cavity and the blood pressure in the cerebral veins will suffice to determine once and for all that the more rapid changes in brain volume are mediated by another mechanism than by the displacement of the cerebrospinal fluid.

In the meantime, I do not wish to deny in the least that there exist conditions under which in a very small and for me imperceptible way, under physiologic circumstances, and in much greater measure in certain pathologic states, even the displacements of the cerebrospinal fluid should be considered in the formation of the movements of the brain. I shall discuss this topic more fully in Chapter 14 of my treatise, and I will develop my views regarding the most essential conditions of normal circulatory relationships in the brain in Chapter 13 ("Movements of the Brain in the Intact Skull").

With respect to the manner in which the crossing of the cerebrospinal fluid from the skull into the spinal canal becomes possible at all, two separate mechanisms have been considered over the course of time, both of which may unquestionably be effective within certain limits; however, both have plainly served as the foundation of multiple, in themselves somewhat exclusive, theories of cerebral movements.

The older of these two theories was essentially anatomical and can be designated as the doctrine of the expansion capacity of the spinal canal. The advocates of this theory, among whom Richet,[44] Ecker,[45] Key, and Retzius[46] deserve mention, emphasize the fact that the cranial cavity does not represent a box with airtight closure all around, but that it freely communicates via the foramen occipitale magnum with the interior cavity of the vertebral column, which, as is generally known, consists of superimposed bony rings linked together by elastic membranes. Moreover, the vertebral column is equipped with both large and small lateral openings, which allow for the passage of the spinal nerves and vertebral vessels, and which are only loosely sealed by funnel-shaped, easily movable elastic membranes.

Richet,[47] who treated this topic in a very respected anatomical work, pointed out that the space remaining between the walls of the foramina intervertebralia and conjugata and the passing nerves and vessels is occupied by a soft, semiliquid fatty tissue similar to that which exists between the dura mater spinalis and the bony walls of the spinal canal. An ever so light pressure exerted from the interior can displace this tissue as easily as if it were a liquid, and Richet showed that when one carefully introduces a finger into the spinal canal, one can observe said fatty tissue protrude from the intervertebral foramina and insert itself into the neighboring tissues. He thus concluded that the spinal cavity in its entire length was offered the latitude for lateral expansion by mediation of these canals.

In Cotugno's work *De ischiade nervosa,*[48] we find note of several facts that are of the greatest consequence for the mechanism of these movements. The deserving Neapolitan anatomist had already observed that, as he states, "the tube of the *dura mater* itself, wherein the spinal cord is enclosed, collects the individual spinal nerves by means of a funnel-shaped or a loose sheath-like attachment. And this same sheath accompanies the nerve up to the place close to its exit from the vertebral canal where it forms a ganglion." After demonstrating the connection of the cavity enclosing the spinal cord with the sheaths of the spinal nerve roots by insufflation of air and by injections of mercury, Cotugno added: "Even though the passage of air and of mercury beyond the ganglion succeeded only under a certain amount of pressure, this pressure was nevertheless very light and in any case not nearly as great as to suggest an obstacle which in living man the spinal vapor (*vapor spinae*)[49] would not be able to overcome."

Key and Retzius[50] in recent years again took up Cotugno's investigations, and for this purpose they used colored liquid. They also noticed that the fluids injected into the subarachnoid spaces penetrated to the bundles of the spinal nerve roots, spread in the ganglion of the posterior root, and also went beyond it. Although, like Cotugno, they did not measure the exact amount of pressure under which they carried out their injections, one can nevertheless discern from their data that they did not exceed the limits of the pressure occurring under natural circumstances in the craniospinal cavity; rather, the authors expressly maintained that only extremely light pressure was required to see the injected fluid penetrate into the nerve bundles and spread between its individual fibers.

In addition to this elasticity of the sheaths accompanying the spinal nerve roots at their exit from the vertebral cavity, and to the facility with which the cerebrospinal fluid spreads within the subarachnoid spaces along the spinal nerves, which alone would suffice to refute the theory of the inelasticity of the cerebrospinal cavity, we must also take into account the mobility of the intervertebral ligaments that easily follow the changing internal pressure. Ecker[51] was the first to observe that the membrana obturatoria posterior (or ligamentum atlanto-occipitale posterius), when exposed, displays rising and sinking motions, of which the first corresponds to expiration, the latter to inspiration.

The configuration of the veins in the skull is, as is generally known, not only different from that in the vertebral canal but also in many ways reversed. While the large venous trunks of the brain, encased in reflections (*Duplicaturen*) of the dura mater, represent broad yet rigid and sparse canals, the venous webs of the vertebral canal are of extremely variable strength and are so numerous that anyone who has ever been involved with injections will have seen the entire interior surface of the vertebral canal covered with a highly dense network of veins. Concentrating on these relationships, Magendie spoke of a mechanism by which the venous vessels of the vertebral cavity promote and mediate the movements of the cerebrospinal fluid.

Thus arose a new theory, which one might call the **doctrine of the repression of venous blood into the spinal blood vessels mediated by the cerebrospinal fluid.**

We need only think of the extraordinary number of veins coating the internal surface of the vertebral canal and consider the thinness of their walls to gain the conviction that these veins must fill up or empty with but minimal pressure variations. Since the vertebral venous webs are not connected directly to the circulation of the central organs of the nervous system, for they empty into the azygous vein and the abdominal veins, they can be viewed as a large reservoir or, better yet, as an elastic cushion surrounding the nerve centers filled with venous blood wherein, under normal circumstances, the very slow-flowing blood accumulates, or from which it exits with the greatest ease, depending on whether, for any reason, the volume of the nerve centers increases or decreases, and the cerebrospinal fluid is driven back and forth accordingly.

Given this, both of the just-discussed mechanisms through which the local variations of the cerebrospinal fluid are mediated are to be regarded only as auxiliary to the concept according to which the overflowing of the said liquid out of the skull into the vertebral canal, and vice versa, would constitute the essential condition for the fluctuating blood content and for the changes in brain volume. Substantially different from this understanding is that which we already found briefly alluded to in Lorry's important treatise *Sur les mouvements du cerveau et de la dure-mère,*[52] in which the author states that **the brain, in the course of its volume increase, could displace the blood from the surrounding veins.**

Later, Cappie[53] put forth the doctrine that in the brain it was not actually the absolute amount of blood that changed, but rather its distribution among the arteries, capillaries, and veins. Thus came into being another new theory, which we can call the theory of the **alternating complementary displacement of the blood between the cerebral veins and the cerebral arteries.** While in this entire theory I hold inadmissible the claim that the absolute blood content of the brain cannot vary at all, I am otherwise of the opinion that the mechanism advocated by Cappie is really the one that is considered most often in the varying circulatory conditions of the brain, and that I believe to have been sufficiently established through my experiments, which will be described in the last chapter of this treatise.

4

Although in our opinion the previously developed considerations should be enough to demonstrate that in the cerebrospinal cavity no great obstacle opposes the variations in volume that the brain, like all organs and parts of the body, must experience under the influence of respiration and cardiac contraction, the incidence of brain movements in the intact skull is nevertheless generally denied by physiologists. The experiments conducted in 1839 by Bourgougnon[54] procure such a semblance of truth to the doctrine denying those movements that since then, most physiologists had accepted it as an established fact. The importance accorded by Longet, Beclard, and others to the teachings of Bourgougnon leads us to discuss the methods of his investigations briefly, and to illuminate the meaning of the conclusions he drew from them.

The apparatus employed by Bourgougnon consisted of a glass tube, which ended at the bottom with a steel screw so that it could be firmly fastened to a hole drilled into the skull by trepanation. Near the middle of the tube there was a spigot and in the lower part (inside the tube) a lever curved at a right angle, which could be moved around a diagonal axis. The horizontal arm of the lever, which could move up and down, was very short and carried a small horizontal plate that protruded from under the steel ending in order to be brought into direct contact with the contents of the skull; the vertical arm (which swung toward the interior wall of the tube when the short lever was raised) did not reach to the level of the spigot.

After the instrument had been applied to the skull of a dog, two thirds of the tube was filled with water. It made no difference in the results of the experiment if the small plate came into contact with the cerebral convolutions covered by dura mater or only by the visceral membrane of the arachnoid, or even directly with tissue that had been freed of both envelopes. If one opened the spigot, one could detect movements of the fluid and oscillations of the lever corresponding to the heartbeat, and one could similarly recognize that the fluid sank during inspiration and rose during expiration. However, if the spigot was shut, the fluid column remained entirely still.

Longet concluded from this experiment that the volume of the brain did not change at all during the phases of respiration. Since, however, he maintained that the brain received less blood during inspiration and at the same time lost more blood through the veins, he believed himself forced to a conciliatory assumption, that during inspiration a **rarefaction** of the brain took place, and during expiration a **compaction.**

Aside from the fact that the hypothesis of such variations in the density of the brain mass is not supported by any evidence and is probably completely superfluous, the only conclusion that might be drawn from Bourgougnon's experiment is that the brain (contrary to Ravina's erroneous assumption) neither visibly pulsates at the points of contact with the inflexible surface of the skull nor presents visible respiratory swings: this latter conclusion disregards the fact that there are indeed flexible areas present within the bony intact skull (such as, for instance, the foramen occipitale magnum) where more or less sizable displacements either of the cerebrospinal fluid or of the brain mass would be conceivable, and which would afford the necessary room to the disputed volume swings of the brain. This possibility could not in any way be discarded by Bourgougnon's experiment, whereas other experiences (specifically the previously mentioned experiment by Ecker with the animal membrana obturatoria posterior) speak for this to a high degree.

If we do not, in spite of this, want to assert unconditionally the real and constant occurrence of intrinsic pulsations and respiratory variations of the brain in the closed skull, this is not because Bourgougnon's experiment excluded this very possibility but because our experiences support the fact that in most cases, specifically in the closed skull, the mentioned movements of the brain mass itself are replaced by another phenomenon: namely, by the alternating dilatation and contraction of the cerebral arteries to the detriment of the venous vessels of the brain that behave in a contrary fashion (Cappie's mechanism, see earlier, p. 15).[55]

However, if we a priori disregard this other modality completely, considering only the possibility of displacements at the flexible areas at the base of the skull, and if we want to be fully clear about what must occur at these areas in the experiments of Bourgougnon and others, then it must be highlighted above all that the two movements that we have so far looked at more closely, namely, the pulsations and the respiratory swings, are not in any way particular only to the brain, but pertain, as we will see directly, to all parts of the body, albeit to different degrees. Furthermore, it is only due to the peculiar conditions brought about by confinement inside the rigid skullcap, which can, however, be re-created artificially for other parts of the body, that these movements turn out to be so marked and extensive within a circumscribed portion of the brain coming to light at the base of a gap in the roof of the skull, whereas at the surface of exposed body parts they are only noticeable with the help of specialized equipment. Given the suggested correspondence, the antagonism that must exist between two or more variably flexible areas of the cranial wall will be obvious to us and can be derived (excepting still the eventuality of Cappie's mechanism) from what happens to the visible movements of the brain when we shut the spigot in Bourgougnon's tube screwed into a skull opening.

In 1846, Piégu had already shown in the course of an experiment that in every part of the body, if placed in the same conditions as the brain, the same volume swings as in the latter become noticeable, too; and similarly, we can eliminate from the brain all semblance of movement when we deprive it of its bony wrapping and observe it in a fully exposed condition.

Thus, indeed, Senac[56] saw that when the entire surface of the brain is exposed, all movement disappears: "qu'on enlève le crâne d'un chien et qu'on mette tout le cerveau à découvert, on n'y verra aucun battement." [Trans.: "If one removes the skull of a dog and uncovers the whole brain, one will not see any pulsation."]

We notice the movements of the brain in an opening of the skull not because they pertain exclusively to this viscus, but because the cerebrospinal cavity, next to the cerebrospinal fluid, represents an apparatus that concentrates at the exposed location of the surface of the brain the sum total of very small and in themselves imperceptible movements that are imparted to this spot from all points of the brain surface. If the cerebrospinal fluid is removed, one can no longer perceive any movement. Thus, Donders, after clearly distinguishing the cerebral movements in the trephined skull of a rabbit, pumped the cerebrospinal fluid out through the ligamentum obturatorium posterius with a very fine syringe and saw as a result that all pulsations and movements stopped immediately, and that instead a movement of the liquid at the place of outflow in the region of the neck commenced. Conversely, if one inserts a forearm into a cylinder and if one closes this off on all sides except for a small opening serving to pour in water, one sees in this opening the same movements appear as in the cerebrospinal fluid of a trephined skull. The apparatus that I constructed and called the **plethysmograph** is based on this very principle and helped me to demonstrate that even in the forearm, aside from the pulsatile variations in volume corresponding to the cardiac contractions, other movements take place that coincide with the respiratory phases so that the forearm experiences an increase in volume with expiration, and a decrease with inspiration.[57]

The plethysmograph essentially represents a reproduction of the fluid-filled box in which the central organs of the nervous system are enclosed; the same mechanism through which the movements of the brain manifest themselves was applied by the plethysmograph for the study of volume changes of the forearm. The only difference here is in the relationship between the mass of the organs and the amplitude of their oscillations, which in the brain, being particularly in its large substance much more richly vascularized, and where the vessels distinguish themselves by the thinness of their walls, turn out to be much more extensive.

Instead of leaving a free opening for communication with the atmosphere in the container into which the forearm is introduced or inserting into this opening a horizontal glass tube so as to observe the variations corresponding to cardiac contractions and respiratory phases, we can seal the opening by means of an elastic membrane, which then will display oscillations very similar to those we observe at the fontanels of children or upon the exposed ligamentum atlanto-occipitale of animals.

Let us now suppose that the forearm is introduced into a cylindrical container such as that of the plethysmograph, but that the container is equipped with two openings, one of which communicates freely with the atmosphere by means of a Bourgougnon glass tube, but the other is closed off by an elastic membrane; it is then clear that the movements of the fluid inside the Bourgougnon tube, where there is less resistance, will manifest themselves more markedly. However, if we close off this tube with a spigot, then the volume oscillations of the forearm will immediately produce distinct swings within the elastic membrane of the other opening, where resistance has now become relatively diminished.

Donders already conducted a similar trial using a rabbit.[58] After prior observation of the movements of the ligamentum atlanto-occipitale in the intact skull, he trephined the skull: the movements of the ligamentum atlanto-occipitale became invisible; instead, they became manifest at the cranial opening where the resistance was lower. However, as soon as the trephined opening was sealed to the air, the movements of the aforementioned ligament resumed.

If one closes the spigot of the Bourgougnon tube, the only possible consequence for the cerebral movements (aside from the still more probable establishment of Cappie's mechanism) will be that while at the opening in the roof of the skull they suddenly stop, they will restart with their previous force in the unquestionably present, flexible sites at the base of the skull.

5

The theory rejecting any movement of the nerve centers in the presence of a closed skull underwent a profound transformation with Donders and his student Berlin, which is all the more noteworthy as it marks a quasi-conciliatory standpoint between the two opposite views strenuously represented in most recent times by Ecker on the one hand and Longet on the other. It is true that the two treatises published simultaneously in 1850 by Berlin[59] and by Donders[60] hold fast to the notion of the inelasticity and rigidity of the cerebrospinal cavity as an uncontested fact, yet they also allow the possibility of variations of the blood content within the closed skull because, according to the authors, the amount of cerebrospinal fluid can increase or decrease in accordance with changes in blood pressure. We want to outline the main features of the data upon which this idea rests, as well as the considerations linked to them by Berlin.

Berlin's experiments demonstrate first of all that the amount of blood in the cranial cavity is variable, that it diminishes with decreased blood pressure and rises with increased blood pressure; further, that when death occurs through slow exsanguination, the decrease in the amount of blood in the cranial cavity is far more marked than with rapid bleeding to death; and that the variable relationship between blood and cerebrospinal fluid can only be recognized after a certain amount of time (following blood loss) has passed, but that, in any case, when there is diminution of the total blood volume, the amount of cerebrospinal fluid increases.

Even though Berlin in no way demonstrated this latter fact rigorously, we nevertheless accept it as established, in the same manner as the others, since the increase of the cerebrospinal fluid in the skull observed with the decrease of the quantity of blood by Berlin could not, even in our estimation, be due to its crossing from the vertebral cavity into the skull, for such a local variation would presume the presence of negative pressure in the cranial space, in which case a much more likely outcome would be marked dilatation of the intracranial veins, rather than the inflow of cerebrospinal fluid. It follows therefore that, in this case, one must indeed hypothesize an increased production of this fluid, and we glimpse in this fact, to be considered as proven, a new mechanism by which the achievement of hyperemic states (or, respectively, anemias) of the brain would also then be possible when the mechanisms otherwise active in such circulatory variations could, for whatever reason, not go into effect.

Regarding the manner in which, when there is increased blood volume of the brain, the increased production of cerebrospinal fluid is achieved, we cannot, however, declare our agreement with Berlin's views. He draws attention to the fact that the high pressure under which the blood flows in the arterial trunks is passed on to the cerebrospinal fluid, which for its part is in contact with the capillaries where blood pressure is lower. He therefore believes that when arterial blood pressure rises, the cerebrospinal fluid, to restore equilibrium, is partially reabsorbed by the capillaries, and that this partial dwindling of cerebrospinal fluid is linked to an increase in the amount of blood circulating in the nerve centers. Were arterial blood pressure to diminish, however, then the amount of cerebrospinal fluid would rise. Even though we accept the principle upon which this theory is based, that between two liquids separated by a membrane and subjected to differential pressures a flow toward the area of lower pressure is set off, we are nevertheless unconvinced by the process hypothesized by Berlin; on the contrary, we are of the opinion that the activity of the lymphatic vessels may play the most important role here.

The investigations published by Donders on the **movements of the brain and the changing blood content, which the vessels of the pia mater can present even in the closed and inextensible skull**, were conducted in the following manner: he drilled a hole in the bone of the skull (using a trephine) and sealed it from the air with a watch crystal through which the surface of the brain could be observed. While on the one hand we wish to highlight the priority of Ravina as the inventor of this method, which in physiology now is incorrectly named for Donders, on the other hand we cannot but recognize that the modification introduced by Donders, namely, the elimination of airspace between the surface of the brain and the glass, constitutes a significant advance and is of great value for the study of the changing circulatory conditions of the brain surface. Yet, the same observation holds true for this procedure as that we have already had to make regarding the experiments of Bourgougnon: while it proves that the brain mass neither visibly pulsates at its points of contact with the inelastic

skull nor undergoes visible respiratory oscillations, it does not rule out the possibility of pulse and respiration swings of the brain volume, for this does not
at all refute the existence of compliant (pliable) spots at the base of the skull
where such movements could very well take place. If one seals the only opening
through which one was able to observe the brain with a transparent and rigid
object, the movements of the hemispheres need not therefore cease, but in this
case they will only be restored to their previous extent at a pliable location of the
cerebrospinal cavity where resistance is relatively lower, unless, prior to trepanation, the mechanism set up by Cappie (see earlier) was already operating instead,
and now again becomes active.

The conclusion drawn by Donders, "that the cerebral movements cannot
take place in a non-compliant skull because the entire cerebrospinal space
is continuously filled, and the amount of blood cannot undergo an instantaneous substantial variation," is in my opinion inadmissible. On the other hand,
I maintain that, just to the contrary, Donders's experiments demonstrate the
possibility and real occurrence of rapid volume changes of the brain in attesting
to the fact that the volume of blood inside the skull is subjected to extremely
rapid variations.

Indeed, Donders saw that when he plugged up the mouth and nose of an animal, the red color of the pia mater intensified within 10 seconds, and with a
microscope he was able to identify the filling up of many small vessels that had
not been visible beforehand. After restoring respiration, this congestion lasted
for a certain amount of time, which varied from 2 to 15 minutes. True, Donders
evidently assumed that the hyperemia just involved the vessels of the pia mater,
and since even this required space, he accepted Berlin's hypothesis that with
each blood pressure variation in the cranial cavity, that following the respiratory
movements as well as the cardiac contractions, the amount of cerebrospinal fluid
must vary accordingly.

One objection arising spontaneously is that the movements of heart and
breath follow each other in such rapid sequence that even if each of these were
to correspond to a variation in the quantity of cerebrospinal fluid, it would be
difficult for us to grasp with our current conceptions such a rapid secretion and
reabsorption of this fluid. Donders, who anticipated this objection, stressed the
large superficial expansion of the brain hemispheres and their rich vasculariza-
tion, which could offset the briefness of the time period within which these phenomena could ensue.

Kussmaul and Tenner[61] also used, for the study of the cerebral circulation,
the method of drilling an opening into the skull and closing it with a watch
crystal. Their observations confirm the results obtained by Donders but are even
more surprising with regard to the rapidity with which the amount of blood
circulating in the nervous centers can change even in the setting of a closed
skull. Indeed, when they laced up then released the carotids in quick succession,
they witnessed the instantaneous filling and emptying of the cerebral vessels in
exactly the same manner, whether the trepanning hole in the skull was open or
closed by a crystal.

Even though these two researchers accepted the Berlin-Donders theory as probable, they admitted nonetheless that they were not granted the opportunity to demonstrate by experiment that, in the rabbit, the rapid variations of the cerebral blood volume were accompanied by an equally rapid, opposite variation of the cerebrospinal fluid.

Rather, and in contrast to the Berlin-Donders theory, they saw that the rabbits who died following ligature of the capital arteries generally displayed less cerebrospinal fluid than other live rabbits, which had been kept in the same position and in which no blood vessels were tied off but where the membrana obturatoria was incised.

Kussmaul and Tenner, from their numerous and extensive experiments, concluded that even in the live animal and in an intact skull, the intracranial blood volume can significantly increase and decrease.

Specifically, a very substantial accumulation of blood in the skull ensued each time the neck arteries were released after previous compression, and the same happened when the neck veins were tied off, especially after concurrent transsection of the two sympathetic cervical trunks.

Anemia of the brain, however, was produced through hemorrhage, or through ligation of the carotids and through electrical stimulation of the vasomotor nerves of the head, and was demonstrable in the small arteries, the capillaries, and the veins.[62]

6

Up until now we have occupied ourselves with the, as it were, macroscopic physiology of the cerebral movements. Now begins, with the employment of the graphic method, the more delicate observation: the comparison of the blood circulation in the brain to that in other parts of the body, the measurement and analysis of the fleeting and complicated phenomena that the naked eye was unable to grasp.

The first experiments to measure the cerebral movements were undertaken by the Italian physician Ravina at the start of this century. To this end, he applied to the skull of a dog a hollow cylinder, inside which a graduated elderberry column, rising and falling like the floating part of a gauge, could follow the movements of the brain. The thin upper end of this column slid along a paper scale, and in this way indicated the parts corresponding to the brain movements. But let us cite verbatim Ravina's own description:

Momentum dimensurus motus cerebri, qui respirationi respondet, usus sum ligneo cylindro superius memorato. Operculo remoto, cylindrum apposui, et firmavi ad oram vulneris, quod in cranio molossi canis institueram. Ex ferro duo parva fila cylindrum tunc secabant in ora ejusdem superiori, ad invicem ita dimota, ut per ipsa columna ex medulla sambuci parata lineae unius diametri moveri commode posset. Iuxta columnam, quae supra memorata fila aliquantisper prominebat, chartam agglutinaveram in plures lineas apprime divisam. Haec columna exili suberis lamina, verticali directione, insistens dimittebatur supra superficiem cerebri, ut per media fila praedicta transiret. . . In validioribus, longioribusque inspirationibus, cum usque ad finem eorundem minueretur volumine cerebrum, ad tres lineas columnam descendere, quandoque conspexi.[63]

[Trans.: To measure the motion of the brain that responds to respiration, I used the wooden cylinder noted above. Having removed the lid I applied the cylinder and pressed it to the mouth of the wound that I had made in the skull of a hunting dog. Two small iron filaments divided the cylinder in its superior opening, which were removed by turns so that thereby the column of elderberry could easily move the filaments by one diameter. Next to the column, from which the above-mentioned filaments protruded a fair amount, I firmly glued a paper chart divided into several lines. This column was released by a thin sheet of cork sitting vertically over the surface of the brain, so that the aforementioned filament crossed in the middle. . . . During more vigorous, prolonged inspirations, at the end of which the brain diminished in volume, the column descended by three lines whenever I watched.]

In Germany in 1855, Bruns,[64] who deserves credit for the first attempt to augment the movements of the brain by means of a lever, undertook human experiments akin to those of Ravina in animals. The observations of this researcher were conducted in a 49-year-old woman who had lost nearly her entire left frontal bone as a consequence of tertiary syphilitic processes. When she introduced herself to Bruns, she presented in the left parietal region a scar as wide as the palm of a hand, beneath which a correspondingly large bony defect could be detected where movements of the brain could be perceived. To measure these, Bruns used a very mobile and light lever, whose shorter arm could be brought into contact with the dura mater by means of a small pad. The second arm, 10 times longer, indicated on a scale graduated in millimeters the value, multiplied by 10, of each brain movement.

In this fashion, he discovered that in a voluntarily protracted expiration the end of the long lever rose by 0.5 to 1.0 mm; with coughing it rose 1.0 to 2.5 mm, and once it even rose 3.0 mm. Deep, prolonged inspiration resulted in the falling of the long arm of the lever by about 0.2 to 0.3 mm below the level of quiet breathing, and a similar, roughly 0.2-mm fall occurred on one occasion during the patient's sleep.

We also wish to make mention here of a study by Hammond[65] in Philadelphia that is, incidentally, of lesser interest as regards its technical aspect.

The study of cerebral movements made a significant advance later on, when for the first time Leyden[66] applied a recording device to the animal skull. To this effect, he used an apparatus patterned after Ludwig's kymograph, which he did

not describe because the data he obtained, of which he only published some fragments, had turned out too imperfectly.

Langlet[67] studied the movements of the fontanels of children, for which he
used a Marey sphygmograph modified in minor ways. Aside from the great difficulty in keeping the head of the child immobilized during the recording, Langlet
found the noise of the clock that set the apparatus in motion very disturbing.
For this latter reason his experiment to study the blood circulation in the brain
during sleep did not succeed, because the children woke up every time the apparatus was set into motion. These unfavorable circumstances led Langlet to dis-
allow that **quiet** breathing movements had any influence on the movements of
the brain; such an influence he found only with forceful breathing, for example,
when the children wept or cried.

Later on the application of the graphic method was attempted with better luck
by myself in conjunction with Prof. Giacomini,[68] and at the same time in Paris
by Salathé and Franck.[69] Shortly thereafter, a treatise with images of brain pulsations was published by Dr. W. Flemming,[70] later followed by a series of observations that I conducted in collaboration with Dr. Albertotti Sr.[71] on a mentally
retarded epileptic patient.[72]

The technological perfecting of the method of continuous recording[73] of the
human pulse in the forearm and in the brain that I had achieved, and the fortunate chance to be able to observe a typical skull defect, allowed me, together
with Dr. De Paoli, to perform such an important series of graphic studies of the
blood circulation in the human brain that in the present work I will barely be
able to take into account similar studies of other researchers and am permitted
to consider almost exclusively my own observations.

NOTES

1. G. Althann: *Beiträge zur Physiologie und Pathologie der Circulation*. I. *Der
   Kreislauf in der Schädelhöhle*. Dorpat, 1871.
2. A. Salathé: *Recherches sur les mouvements du cerveau*. Paris, 1877.
3. A. Mosso: *Introduzione ad una serie di esperienze sui movimenti del cervello neel'
   uomo*. Archivio per le scienze mediche, I, fasc. 2, 1876.
4. C. Plinii: *Historia naturalis,* lib. VII, cap viii. Augustae Taurinorum, 1831, vol. III,
   p. 92.
5. Subsequent Latin citations will be reproduced as included in the original text,
   together with English translations. French quotes are usually translated in the
   body of the text without the original citation.
6. Galeni: *Opera, ex versione latina*. Venetiis, 1562, pp. 124, 250, 307.
7. *Oeuvres d*'Oribase par Bussemaker et Daremberg. Paris, 1857, vol. III, p. 307.
8. Ibid., vol. III, p. XIX.
9. G. Fallopii: *Observationes anatomicae*. Venetiis, 1562, p. 221.
10. A. Vesalii: *Anatomicarum Fallopii observationem examen*. Hanoviae, 1600, p. 258.

11. Schlichting: *De motu cerebri*. Mémoires de mathématique et physique. Acad. des sciences des savants étrangers. Paris, 1750, T. I, p. 113.

12. A. Pacchioni: *Opera*. Romae, 1741, pp. 92 and 136.

13. G. Baglivi: *Opera*. Lugduni, 1714, p. 279.

14. Lamure: *Mémoire sur la cause des mouvements du cerveau qui paraissent dans l'homme et dans les animaux trépanés*. Histoire de l'Académie royale des sciences. 1753, p. 541.

15. Haller: *Elementa physiologiae*.Lausanne, 1762, IV, p. 173.

16. Haller: *Mémoires sur la nature sensible et irritable des parties du corps animal*. Lausanne, 1756, p. 31.

17. Lorry: *Sur les mouvements du cerveau et de la dure-mère*. Mémoires de mathématique et de physique. Paris, 1760, T. III, p. 305.

18. Cotugno: *De ischiade nervosa*. Viennae, 1770, p. 17.

19. Cotugno, 21.

20. Portal: *Cours d'anatomie médicale*. Paris, 1804, T. IV, p. 66.

21. Richerand: *Nouveaux éléments de physiologie*. Paris, 1749, p. 206.

22. Senac: *Traité de la structure du coeur*. Paris, 1749, p. 206.

23. Burdach: *Bau und Leben des Gehirns*. Leipzig, 1826, p. 32.

24. Aside from the numerous experiments published in his *Mémoires sur la nature sensible*, Haller, foreseeing that objection as it were, wrote the following words in his treatise: "Je vis ce mouvement alternatif que Schlichting avait observé: le cerveau montait dans l'expiration, descendait dans l'inspiration. Ce seul mouvement m'a fait faire plus de trente expériences avec M. Walsdorff, qui les a publiées depuis la première impression de ce Mémoire" (p. 29). [Trans.: "I saw this alternating motion that Schlichting had observed: the brain rose in expiration, sunk in inspiration. This motion alone has caused me to perform more than thirty experiments with M. Walsdorff who has published them since the first printing of this Memoir"].

25. Ravina: *Specimen de motu cerebri*. Mémoires de l'Académie des sciences de Turin. 1811, p. 70.

26. Op. cit., p. 75.

27. Trans.: Vitalism holds that living organisms are fundamentally different from inanimate matter because they contain some nonphysical element, or vital "spirit." The French physiologist Xavier Bichat was one of the numerous figures who argued that living organisms possessed vital properties that could not be reduced to their inorganic constituents.

28. Magendie: *Recherches sur le liquide céphalo-rachidien ou cérébro-spinal*. Paris, 1842.

29. Magendie in a note wrote the following: "Having not found the leisure to search in the ancient or the modern authors for what has been written about the liquid that is the special topic of this work, and since—to be honest—*this kind of work for me has no appeal*, I have asked my former student and collaborator, Dr. Jodin, to be kind enough to fill in for me" (Ibid. p. 138).

30. Jodin: *Recherches historiques sur le liquide céphalo-rachidien*. Cited by Magendie, in Ibid. p. 138.

31. Schlichting, op. cit., p. 123.

32. Lamure, op. cit., p. 567.

33. On this matter Lorry expressed himself as follows: "Although the forces of the blood upon the brain may rarely produce a movement in the parts of the brain contained within the skull, as long as the bony case is intact, there are certainly cases when the effort of the blood toward the head is considerably augmented, where I am convinced that a movement within the head can be produced" (Op. cit., 312). This citation may serve as rectification of what Longet, in his *Traité de Physiologie*, p. 319, during his otherwise very thorough historical discussion of cerebral movements, stated about Lorry, and of what Colin and other French authors have alleged.

34. Fabre: *Essais sur différents points de physiologie.* 1770.

35. A. Monro: *Beobachtungen über die Structur und die Functionen des Nervensystems.* Translation by Soemmering. Leipzig, 1787.

36. Abercrombie: *Pathologische und practische Untersuchungen über die Krankheiten des Gehirns und des Rückenmarkes.* Translated from English by Busch. Bremen, 1829.

37. Kellie: Transactions of the medico-chirurgical Society of Edinburgh, vol. I (cited by Abercrombie).

38. Bergmann: *Kreislauf,* in Wagner's Handwörterbuch der Physiologie. Vol. II, p. 300. Braunschweig, 1844.

39. J. Hamernik: *Physiologisch-pathologische Untersuchungen über die Verhältnisse des Kreislaufes in der Schädelhöhle.* Vierteljahrschrift f. pract. Heilkunde, published by the Faculty of Medicine of Prague. Vol. XVII.

40. Op. cit., p. 395.

41. Burow: *Beobachtungen über die Krankheiten des cerebralen Blutkreislaufes und den Zusammenhang zwischen Hirn- und Herzleiden.* German [translation] by Posner. Leipzig, 1847.

42. Kussmaul und Tenner: *Untersuchungen über Ursprung und Wesen der fallsuchtartigen Zuckungen bei der Verblutung.* Moleschott's *Untersuchungen,* III, p. 56.

43. Th. Ackermann: *Untersuchungen über den Einfluss der Erstickung auf die Menge des Blutes im Gehirn und in den Lungen.* Virchow's Archiv, XV, 1858, p. 401.

44. Richet: *Traité pratique d'anatomie médico-chirurgicale.* 3. edition. Paris. 1866.

45. Ecker: *Physiologische Untersuchungen über die Bewegungen des Gehirns und Rückenmarkes.* Stuttgart, 1843.

46. Key and Retzius: *Studien in der Anatomie des Nervensystems und des Bindegewebes.* Stockholm, 1875.

47. Op. cit., p. 284.

48. Op. cit., ch. XXIV, p. 39.

49. In his treatise, Cotugno at times used the inappropriate term *vapor* instead of *humor* to designate the cerebrospinal fluid. Yet, as we saw on p. 6, he himself expressly insisted that this was not vapor but water, in other words a liquid that can form droplets, the existence of which his experiments had demonstrated even in the live animal.

50. Op. cit.

51. Op. cit., p. 191.

52. Mémoires de mathématique et de physique. Paris, 1760, T. III.

53. J. Cappie: *Ueber die Beziehung des Schädelinhaltes zu dem Drucke der Atmosphäre.* Edinb. Med. Journal, XX, p. 105, 1874 (Schmidt's Jahrbücher, 1875, 15. März, p. 131).

54. Bourgougnon: Dissertation inaugurale. Paris, 1838, cited by Longet, *Traité de physiologie*, p. 311.

55. See p. 15.

56. Senac: *Traité de la structure du coeur*. Paris, 1749, Vol. II, p. 206.

57. A. Mosso: *Sopra un nuovo metodo per scrivere i movimenti dei vasi sanguigni nell' uomo*. Regia Accademia delle scienze di Torino, vol. XI, 1875. This work discussed in brief the history of studies of respiratory and pulsatile movements of the extremities.

58. Donders: *Die Bewegungen des Gehirns und die Veränderungen der Gefässfüllung der Pia mater auch bei geschlossenem, unausdehnbarem Schädel, unmittelbar beobachtet*. Schmidt's Jahrbücher, 1851, Vol. 69, p. 17.

59. Berlin: *Untersuchungen über den Blutumlauf in der Schädelhöhle*. Schmidt's Jahrbücher, 1851, Vol. 69, p. 14.

60. Donders: *Die Bewegungen des Gehirns und die Veränderungen der Gefässfüllung der Pia mater auch bei geschlossenem, unausdehnbarem Schädel, unmittelbar beobachtet*. Schmidt's Jahrbücher, 1851, Vol. 69, p. 16.

61. Kussmaul and Tenner, op. cit., p. 49.

62. While, as noted earlier, we do not doubt the authenticity of the fact observed by Berlin, we believe we must account for the contradictory results of Kussmaul and Tenner with the assumption that during these authors' experiments, other, not more closely illuminated circumstances would have been at work.

63. Op. cit., p. 74.

64. Bruns: *Die chirurgischen Krankheiten und Verletzungen des Gehirns und seiner Umhüllungen*. Tübingen, 1854, p. 601.

65. W. Hammond: *Sleep and its derangements*. Philadelphia, 1869, p. 317.

66. W. Leyden: *Beiträge und Untersuchungen zur Physiologie und Pathologie des Gehirns*. Virchow's Archiv, 1866, Vol. 37, p. 519.

67. J. B. Langlet: *Études critiques sur quelques points de la physiologie du sommeil*. Paris, 1872.

68. C. Giacomini e A. Mosso: *Esperienze sui movimenti del cervello nell' uomo*. Archivio per le scienze mediche, I, fasc. 3, 1876.

69. Salathé: *Recherches sur les mouvements du cerveau*. Paris, 1877.

70. W. Flemming: *The motions of the brain*. Glasgow Medical Journal, July 1877.

71. Albertotti e Mosso: *Osservazioni sui movimenti del cervello di un idiota epilettico*. R. Accademia di Medicina di Torino, 1877.

72. See, "Thron," Chapter 1.2., p. 31.

73. A. Mosso: *Die Diagnostik des Pulses*. Leipzig, 1879.

Notes Concerning the Disease States of the Three Subjects in Whom the Conditions of the Blood Circulation in the Brain Were Studied

The observations about the cerebral blood circulation discussed in the present text were carried out primarily on three human individuals suffering from acquired loss of cranial substance. Two of them are still alive and enjoy a relative state of well-being. The third subject, an 11- to 12-year-old boy named Giovanni Thron, died a few months after we observed him, and approximately 10 years after the trauma that resulted in the ectopy of his brain. For the first two subjects I also provide, aside from their medical history notes, the portraits executed on the basis of their photographs (Plates 1.1 and 1.2).

§. 1.1

Catherina X., 37 years old, a farmer's wife, entered the Syphilocomium of San Lazzaro in Turin in June of 1875. Married since age 18, she had given birth to six children and had always been well. During her last pregnancy, her husband infected her with syphilis. While the vaginal chancre was left to heal spontaneously, no general treatment was initiated. The woman delivered in August 1866 and nursed the child herself. This child died of measles in January 1868.[1] Two years later symptoms of generalized syphilis, tertiary to be exact, appeared in the woman (whether in the interim the usual secondary symptoms failed to appear or only passed unnoticed remains uncertain): Violent headaches developed in the frontal region and swellings (probably gummatous skin lesions)

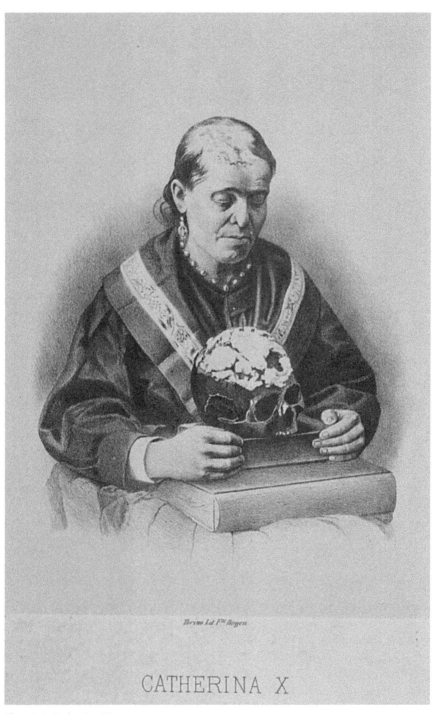

CATHERINA X

Plate 1.1 Catherina X.

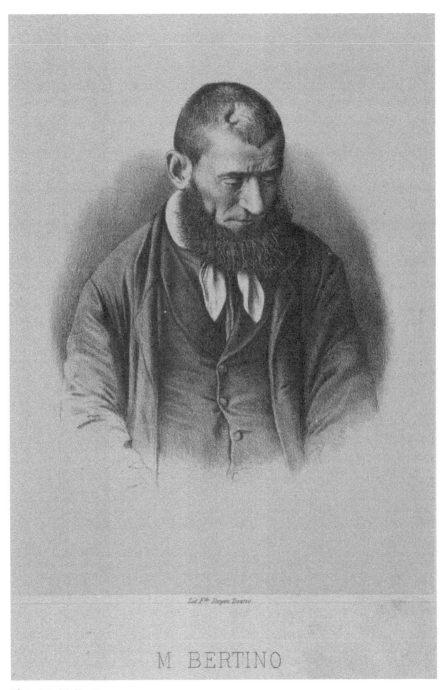

Lit. F.lli Doyen Torino

M BERTINO

Plate 1.2 M. Bertino.

appeared in different parts of her body, which ulcerated and left deep scars. Treatment with potassium iodide was carried out.[2] Regression of all syphilitic symptoms ensued. In the following year, however, the gummatous tumors reappeared. In 1869, the patient was admitted to San Giovanni General Hospital in Turin, and during the following year to San Lazzaro Hospital, where she remained for 6 months. Seemingly cured, she returned to the countryside and found herself to be quite well throughout the next 2 years. After this period her headaches recurred, and at the same time new gummatous formations appeared simultaneously on the hard palate, the soft palate, and the nose, which quickly ulcerated and completely destroyed the vomer, the bony palate, and the nasal cartilage. In August of 1872, the patient was readmitted to San Lazzaro Hospital where for the fourth time she underwent internal treatment with potassium iodide together with topical mercury applications. After she had felt reasonably well for a period of time, a swelling appeared at the jugular notch, which ruptured and progressed to ulcer formation together with decay of the underlying bone. In spite of all therapeutic efforts, her headaches also resumed, limited to the frontal region where initially one nodule, and later, on both sides, two more became evident. As the superficial soft tissues fell victim to ulcerative destruction, the middle portion of the frontal bone was largely exposed. It was in this condition, extremely emaciated and plagued by ongoing diarrhea, nocturnal fever, and sleeplessness, that on June 22 the patient was admitted to San Lazzaro Hospital for the last time.

While the patient's overall condition, after implementation of the most pressing indications, improved rapidly, Prof. Giacomini soon thought about the most expedient way to remove the entire necrotic portion of the skullcap. He pierced the middle of the frontal bone with a Nélaton surgical rongeur[3] and gradually reached the internal layer, which was easier to breach. As soon as this was done, a substantial quantity of pus emerged, which revealed a pulsatory motion in the opening of the skull. Within a few days a portion of the dura mater, the width of a coin, was exposed. Its surface was covered with very vascular granulations, which bled at the slightest touch, and which showed distinct pulsations synchronous with cardiac systole.

Just after the operative interventions described previously were finished, we began our experiments with the application of a recording apparatus.

To the extent that the cranial breach became wider with the removal of necrotic bone fragments, the movements of the *dura mater* and the brain became more and more indistinct. The patient lost, little by little, the entire *pars squamosa* of the frontal bone and a large part of the parietal bones. We preserved the detached fragments and later on cemented them together according to their natural position. When we had the patient photographed, we had her hold the resected portion thus reassembled into a whole, and as a result she is depicted in the photograph with a large piece of her own skull in her hand (see Plate 1.1).[4]

The patient did not want to return to her husband any more and was hired as a nursing attendant in one of our hospitals. I recently saw her again. She told me that she was feeling well, and I could verify that the process of ossification was expanding rapidly in various places so that the scar had become hard and inflexible.

§. 1.2

Giovanni Thron, from the region of Pinerolo,[5] was an 11-year-old boy afflicted with idiocy and epilepsy, who had pleasing facial features and beautifully shaped, symmetric body anatomy. He was barely 18 months old when he suffered, subsequent to a fall from a high place, a severe injury in the right temporoparietal area, which healed leaving a scar on his skin and significant loss of substance in the wall of his skull.

According to the sparse anamnestic data we were able to gather, it appeared that after the trauma approximately 1½ years had passed until the first cerebral symptoms of any consequence manifested themselves.

Epileptic attacks, initially epileptiform, later on full fledged, did not appear until the third year of life, and over the course of time, very alarming maniacal symptoms appeared along with these attacks, which persuaded the parents to send the boy to the insane asylum in Turin.[6]

We omit the evolving course of the illness up to the point when we became acquainted with Thron as an imbecilic epileptic patient in the insane asylum.

The intelligence sphere of the patient now was solely limited to ideas connected to the most pressing bodily needs. Yet his memory had preserved at least traces of some concepts of a higher order, because, for example, in response to questions directed at him, he often replied with the following sentence: *veui andà à l'école* ("I want to go to school").[7]At other times he replied with the sound *Mondon*, the significance of which we were unable to elicit.

I observed him oftentimes when he played in the garden and never noticed any anomaly in his movements.

One day, when he did not want to follow me from the garden into his room, I took his hat from his head. He ran after me with a miserable face and in a plaintive, almost weeping voice repeated several times these words: *veui ma calotte* ("I want my cap").

Whenever he could escape the attention of the attendants, he greedily devoured the most revolting things.

Epileptic fits were preceded by a state of agitation during which he became loud and obnoxious. His shouting announced an impending fit, and the attendants then came running to take him to an appropriate place before the attack broke out.

At the time we started our experiments (in the spring of 1877), the boy presented with a defect of the skull in his temporal and parietal areas, bridged by otherwise normal skin but which in the middle was marked by a longitudinal scar. This defect of the bone was of elliptical shape and directed from an inferoposterior position to an anterior superior one. Its longest diameter measured 70 mm, the widest diameter 35 mm. The scar running from one end of the defect to the other in the direction of its longitudinal diameter was about 6 to 7 mm wide and completely hairless.

In the area of the bony defect one could clearly distinguish the pulsations and other movements of the brain.

When the skin sank in, one could discern that the defect was of shallow depth; if one also pushed on the area rather firmly with one's fingers, the scar membrane felt very resistant and no symptoms of cerebral pressure appeared.

In August, while I was away from Turin, the boy took ill with gastroenteritis with extremely profuse diarrhea, which affected his otherwise robust constitution so severely that he succumbed to acute anemia on October 29. During this terminal illness and until the final days of his life, his epileptic fits had neither weakened nor diminished in frequency.

During the inspection of the skull, prepared by Prof. Giacomini, we found the defect to be covered by a tough fibrous membrane, to the exterior surface of which the epidermis (together with the scar) adhered firmly. On the inside this membrane was melded together with the meninges, which themselves clung fast to the cerebral convolutions. The latter had atrophied over a somewhat larger surface than that over which the bony defect extended.

The middle portion of the atrophic area fell into the posterior end of the horizontal branch of the Sylvian fissure. Expanding superiorly from there, the atrophy affected the anterior part of the lower parietal convolution (*lobulus supra-marginalis*) and ended in the middle part of the *gyrus parietalis ascendens*. Inferiorly, the posterior ends of the three gyri temporo-sphenoidales and part of the posterior portion of the *gyrus parietalis inferior s. angularis* had succumbed to atrophy.

§. 1.3

Michele Bertino was a peasant of sturdy build, 37 years old, born at Varicella in the province of Turin.

On July 30, 1877, as he stood below the bell tower of his village, a brick that had slipped from the hands of a mason working near the roof fell on his head. Under the impact of this 3-kg mass dropped from a height of 14 m, Bertino fell to the ground unconscious. The surgeon, Mr. Ferrero, who had to treat him later on, wrote to me that soon after the accident Bertino was picked up and that he went, propped up by the parish priest, to the latter's residence where he was laid on a bed; during this time he reportedly did not in the least lose either speech or the memory of what had occurred. Bertino, on the other hand, claimed to have retained no memory of these happenings and, what is more, claimed not even to remember the blow he suffered and maintained that he regained consciousness only half an hour later. The last he was able to recall of the previous time period related to the moment immediately before the blow: He remembered well that he was standing under the bell tower, watching a comrade who was soaking bricks in water; he himself waited there just to place the bricks into the basket afterward. There followed a moment of darkening, as it were, and when Bertino regained consciousness, he was surprised to see himself lying on a bed with the surgeon holding up a pocket watch and asking him to state what the time was. The patient added that since that moment, and also during his dressing change, he had always been alert and conscious. And indeed, his precise remembrance shed light on various circumstances, also corroborated by the surgeon and by other witnesses.

The crushed laceration, which the fallen mass had generated on the upper part of the forehead, was shaped like an irregular triangle 7 cm long and 4 cm wide and was accompanied by a comminuted fracture of the skull bone. The surgeon who took charge of treating him pulled out of the wound after a few hours several pieces of brick, one of which was about the size of a hazelnut. He also removed from it a piece of hat, the size of a coin of 5 centimes (25 mm in diameter), and approximately seven bony fragments that belonged in part to the outer and in part to the vitreous table of the cranial wall. Bleeding was not inconsiderable. After careful irrigation of the wound, one could see at its base, according to the information provided by the surgeon, the dura mater damaged by penetrating bone splinters and pulsating because of the cerebral movements. Bertino asserted that voluntary movement and sensation of his limbs and of his entire body, just like his mind, remained always perfectly unimpaired.

His very simple treatment consisted of dousings and ablutions with lukewarm phenyl acid water and of continuous application of an ice bag to the site of the skull fracture.

The inflammatory reaction at the surface remained very limited even though there was rather profuse purulence in the deeper parts.

Of the medical history communicated to me by surgeon Ferrero, I emphasized among the more noteworthy details the circumstance that Bertino, upon trying to get up for the first time after having been bedridden for several days, fell to the ground and hit his head against the wall.

Since that time, the surgeon, in accordance with the patient's wish, had to discontinue his daily visits. Then, on two occasions, as Mr. Ferrero indicated, it happened that pus accumulated between the hard meninges and the roof of the skull and gave rise to symptoms of cerebral pressure, which, however, with the institution of appropriate treatment measures abated very soon.

On August 9, surgeon Ferrero removed by means of a dressing forceps a necrotic shred of the dura mater, which had until then plugged the cranial defect; on this occasion, he indicated that after careful cleansing of the wound, the brain mass became very clearly visible and, within it, there was a loss of tissue the size of a hazelnut.

In order to approximate the edges of the skin laceration he applied a suture; toward the end of August he withdrew from the wound edges two further bone splinters.

After the patient had been on bedrest for 24 days, he got up and went to the nearby village of Lanzo, where the local hospital physician examined him. Later on, he consulted the physician at Fiano (another village in the vicinity of

Varicella) for the same purpose. It was only on the pressing advice of all these physicians that Bertino decided to go to Turin.

On September 27, about 2 months after his injury, he was admitted to the local general hospital (San Giovanni). He presented with, on the right side of the skull and on the upper part of the forehead, about 1 cm from the vertical midline of the latter, a continuous separation of the cranial skin and the skull bone of irregular rounded shape and about 25 mm in diameter. The bone defect must have been, I presumed, in close proximity to the coronal suture since it was about 25 mm away from the line connecting the two tubercles on the exterior surface of the zygomatic process. The skin adhered to the entire circumference of the cranial defect, which presented a funnel-shaped floor of a depth of about 3 cm. This indentation was clad with a vivid red membrane with rather flat, small, fleshy warts. If one let the patient lie on his back with his head held horizontally, the indentation of the skull decreased by so much that it corresponded to only a shallow depression of approximately 5 mm in depth. When the patient was in a sitting or upright position, the floor of this depression revealed pulsations that coincided temporally with the radial pulse.

In order to measure the volume of the wound, I poured lukewarm water into it from a graduated glass cylinder and found that to fill up the hollow area, 5 cm^3 of water was required, with the patient in a sitting position and at rest. Since about 4 hours had passed since the last dressing, a quantity of pus not more precisely determinable had accumulated at the base of the wound, which would have to be added to the 5 cm^3 since I did not remove it. However, I did not consider this to be of further importance because the extent of the wound usually fluctuated, for reasons we would later learn.

Secretion of pus was substantial, and if one did not prevent this accumulation of pus in the hollowing of the skull, it caused the patient to experience a sensation of weight in his head.

The patient got out of bed every day and walked continuously about the halls and in the garden. Dr. De Paoli, who oversaw his treatment, noted in his patient history that Bertino did not display any impairment of performance as to intelligence, speech, memory, mobility, or sensation; however, he did show a certain disturbance of the emotional sphere, for his facial features always conveyed an expression of mistrust and anxiety.

Bertino remained at the general hospital only for about a month, and it was during the last week of his stay there that I was able to make, at the invitation of Dr. De Paoli and in conjunction with him, the observations to be discussed later. These were interrupted by the sudden departure of the patient, who insisted on leaving the hospital in order to return to his village and his family.

About 18 months later I wrote to Bertino at Varicella and asked him to come to Turin because I wished to see him. He obeyed my request right away, and when he paid me a visit on March 27, 1879, he told me that he had felt perfectly well during the entire time. A month after his discharge from the hospital he already felt able to provide by his own labor for the livelihood of his family, which consisted of his wife and two children, and he thus took charge of his farming activities. In doing so, he had experienced no difficulties other than noticing that "his brain would rise up" when he made an effort or when he leaned forward.

The scar showed a depression with a longitudinal diameter of approximately 25 mm, directed from the exterior rim of the orbits toward the anterior end of the sagittal suture; the width of the depression was 20 mm. These measurements were made at the floor of the depressed scar; however, its borders were not vertical but somewhat sloping from the periphery toward the middle (in the shape of a trough) and thus the circumference at the level of the skin surface was greater than the one indicated. The depth of the depression (i.e., the vertical distance of its base from the level of the outermost rim) amounted to 5 mm. The floor was smooth and hard and, when pressed, offered a resistance as though there were bones present; yet one is obviously dealing merely with a fibrous scar since during a deep expiration, as we would see, it could rise and pulsate.

Incidentally, as to the patient's statement regarding his complete and uninterrupted euphoria since his hospital discharge, there was nonetheless, as per his further and more precise communications, some qualification to be made in this respect. Indeed, in April 1878 he experienced a kind of "fainting" spell. In the middle of the night his wife, who slept next to him, noticed that he was breathing noisily. She called out to him in order to wake him but became aware that he had lost consciousness and speech. After a few minutes he regained his senses; however, he felt weary and beaten down, with a sensation of lassitude and pain in his arms and legs.

Bertino repeatedly assured me that when he worked he did not feel the least deficit in performance capacity that would remind him of the grave injury he had suffered. However, in his personality he noted this one change: namely, that he had become much more timid; while in the past he had been bold, had liked to meddle in other people's dealings, and had even started fights on his own account, now he avoided the company of his comrades out of fear that some evil might befall him again. He was afraid of everything.

His portrait, which I provide here (Plate 1.2), was created based on a photograph I had taken of Bertino at his last visit, approximately a year and a half following his injury.

During the final observation I made of him at that time, the resistance of the scar proved to be so much greater that even with the application of a very sensitive double recording cylinder, one could not register any pulsation in the skull defect when Bertino remained completely still. It was only during ample respiratory movements that the level of the scar changed and that fluctuations became visible in the recording.

NOTES

1. Trans.: We use the date cited in Mosso's earlier Italian version. In the German version, the date is 1878, which is obviously incorrect given the chronological context.

2. Trans.: Potassium iodide in oral and topical formulations was considered effective against the tertiary stage of syphilis.
3. Trans.: Instrument designed by Auguste Nélaton (1807-1873), personal surgeon to Napoleon III.
4. Trans.: It is unclear whether Mosso was aware of the risk of infection he would incur handling gummatous syphilitic lesions, which can harbor the spirochete. He himself developed locomotor ataxia in 1904.
5. Trans.: A Piedmontese town, not far from Turin.
6. Trans.: Historically, epileptic patients were confined with the mentally ill, but it was only from the late 18th century on that they became the object of systematic medical attention. The separation of epileptic patients in special wards became established procedure around the middle of the 19th century. This was based on the prevailing belief that epilepsy was contagious, and that the witnessing of an epileptic attack might suffice to propagate the disease.
7. Trans.: The patient is speaking a Piedmontese dialect.

Description of the Equipment Used to Record the Pulse of the Brain and of Other Parts of the Body

§. 2.1

The transmission of movement through air using Buisson's paired tambours (more generally known by the name of Marey's) provides, up to the present, the simplest and safest way to reproduce the movements of the pulse at a distance without altering their contour too much.

The experiments I did using other methods to observe the blood circulation in the brain have shown me that the transmission of the brain's movements through a fluid encounters resistances too great and renders the pressure inconstant. The process one might wish to consider first, that is, the direct application of a light lever to the pulsating part of the brain, would certainly be the simplest of all, but in reality it proved to be impracticable because the inevitable displacements of the head made uncertain, and even downright impossible, the continuous registration of the phenomena whose prolonged continuous tracking was essentially at stake.

During the first series of observations, which I performed in conjunction with Dr. Giacomini on Catherina X., we used the Marey *tambour explorateur* connected to a levered barrel.

Since this is a device used on a daily basis by clinicians and physiologists, I will omit its description and refer those who wish to study it more closely to the work of Marey,[1] where the construction of this apparatus is delineated in detail. I will note that the outer wooden bell was fastened to the head in such a way that its rim rested at two opposite points on the firm bony edge of the skull defect, while the knob of the tambour remained above the pulsating surface in the air. The bell was fastened to the head with a cruciate band, and by turning the upper screw the barrel was gradually lowered until its knob lightly touched the spot on the base of the skull defect where the pulsations of the brain appeared most distinctly. The movements of the brain were transmitted to the knob and to the air contained within the barrel, through which they were transferred to the recording cylinder; the lever of the latter recorded them on the blackened paper of the rotating kymograph drum.

During these first studies, we encountered great technical difficulties and were soon discouraged by the additional failure of experiments we had done using other methods. Since time was of the essence, we decided in favor of the cardiograph, in spite of the great disadvantage that this apparatus contains an internal spring, which, because of its resistance, made the pulsations less distinct. Among various difficulties, it is enough to mention that the transmission of the cerebral movements occurred through the mediation of the thickened, granulation-studded *dura mater*, and this in the midst of a wound surface encircled by necrotic bone and thick hair, which we did not want to cut out of consideration for the patient.

The apparatus we used with Dr. Albertotti on Johann Thron was much simpler. We applied a circular gutta percha plate, 4 mm thick and 12 cm in diameter, in a slightly warmed state to the skull after the hair near the scar was shaved off, so that the plate clung snugly to the scar surface and after cooling remained modeled accordingly. The center of the gutta percha plate thus fashioned, we curved it into a dome of sufficient height, so that even with the strongest bulging of the brain the scar could not touch its sides. At the front of the dome I attached a small glass tube 6 cm in length and 6 mm in diameter. To retain during the individual experiments a completely airtight fit between the rim of the gutta percha mold and the area of the skull defect and to keep it fastened to the latter, the mold was heated over an alcohol lamp before each application.

§. 2.2

The pulse tracings obtained by this process were much better than those obtained on Catherina X. because the previously described installation excluded the resistance of the elastic membrane and the stylus located in the Marey *explorateur à tambour*, or cardiograph.

It happened by chance that the individual patients whose nosographic notes were provided in the preceding chapter presented themselves to me one after another under circumstances that became increasingly favorable for the recording of the cerebral movements, so that in the end Bertino, for a period of time, embodied the ideal of a cranial lesion most aptly suited for this purpose. Indeed, I believe it would have been difficult to produce intentionally in animals a cranial defect more profitably designed for this, because when the skull is trephined, as Mr. Salathé[2] correctly pointed out, one often encounters an insurmountable obstacle to the recording of the cerebral movements. The brain, through its swelling, comes into contact with the skull wall and plugs the opening created by the trepan so that after the experiment has barely begun and a few pulsations have been very clearly recorded, these gradually weaken and finally disappear altogether. If in such cases one unscrews the tube inserted into the skull, one discovers that the brain has herniated though the skull defect, protruding from its border and completely obstructing the opening. Such a problem could not happen with Bertino, since in his case there was in the brain an indentation of 5 cm³ underneath the skull defect, which even with the most significant increases in brain volume was not completely filled up.

Since Bertino's 20-mm-wide cranial breach was positioned near the brain and had smooth edges, to close the defect it was sufficient to apply a gutta percha plate equipped with a glass tube at its center, which connected the air within the cerebral indentation to the recording barrel $F\,G$ in Fig. 2.1. One had only to heat the edges of this plate lightly, or coat its inferior surface with grease, to get it to adhere tightly to the skin so that no air could escape.

This very simple device, which served admirably to record the pulsations of the brain and its slight variations in volume, was, however, inadequate for experiments during which there were more significant increases in volume. Thus, we shall see, for instance, that under the influence of amyl nitrite and during other cerebral congestions, the membrane of the recording cylinder is raised up so high that the transcription lever no longer touches the cylinder at all. Even people only somewhat familiar with such experiments are well aware that in such cases one must neither move the instrument nor lower the lever nor carry out other types of manipulations that would distort the recordings and the graphic mechanisms, because otherwise, later on, when the brain volume decreases again, one can no longer reproduce the original conditions of the experiment.

To avoid this problem and record the brain movements under constant pressure without at the same time depriving myself of the possibility of measuring the extent of the variations in cerebral volume with relative precision, I attached the tube connected to the cylinder to two Müllerian valves, as is shown in Fig. 2.1.

When the volume of the brain increased and thus the pressure in the system of tubes A and B rose, an air bubble escaped from the vessel D. On the other hand, when the pressure sank, as happened during a decrease of brain volume, an air bubble penetrated into vessel E from the exterior. I could count the air bubbles and later calculate accordingly the volume correlated to this sum. Most of the time, however, it was not even necessary that I myself or an assistant be occupied with the direct counting of air bubbles, because each time the escape and the entry of air bubbles conveyed a vibration to all the air of the system which left a visible trace in the recording.

§. 2.3

I have always recorded the pulse of the forearm with my hydrosphygmograph. This instrument was all the more helpful to me in the comparative study of the circulatory phenomena in the human brain and forearm since, with it, the

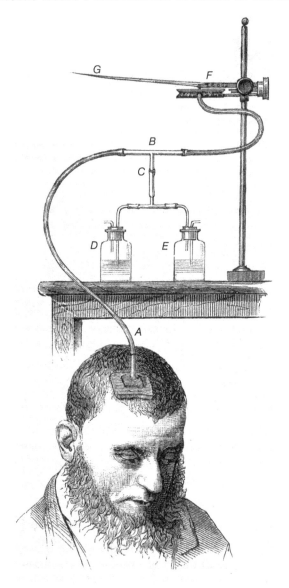

Figure 2.1 Arrangement of the instrument used on Bertino for the recording of the cerebral pulse.

conditions of the experiment and the method of recording for both body parts were the same (Fig. 2.2).

 The hydrosphygmograph consists of a cylindrical glass container *A B*, similar to the glass cylinder of my plethysmograph.[3] I introduce the forearm into the container and close the latter by means of an elastic rubber sleeve *A*, the same as I do using the plethysmograph. The apparatus is suspended from the ceiling of the room to eliminate the harmful influence of involuntary movements. To suspend it, I use an iron chain *H* and attach the apparatus with a small metallic hook to its links. Thereafter, the container is filled with tepid water up to the lower rim of the more than 20-mm-wide lateral tubule *B*. With each cardiac contraction and subsequent inflow of a wave of blood into the forearm there ensues an increase in its volume, which raises the water level in tubule *B*. As a result, the air above it is slightly compressed, and this movement is transmitted via an elastic rubber tube to a Marey tambour *F*, whose lever *N* records the individual pulsations onto the coated paper of a rotating cylinder.

Without this new sphygmograph, it would not have been possible for me to compare the form of the cerebral pulse with that of the forearm on a continuing basis. I have been able to establish these newly observed circulatory phenomena in human subjects essentially thanks to this continuous registration method; the value of these observations is based on the very nature of the procedure I used for the simultaneous recording of the cerebral and the forearm pulse for these two body parts.

Indeed, if one introduces the forearm into the glass cylinder of the hydrosphygmograph and fills the cylinder with water, that part of the body represents an organ submerged in liquid and enclosed within a stiff-walled cavity, just like the brain, which is bathed by the cerebrospinal fluid and enclosed in the cranial cavity. The concordance is complete. The opening of the hydrosphygmograph, where the changes in volume of the forearm are visible, corresponds to the loss of substance of the skull wall, which we connect to the recording cylinder.

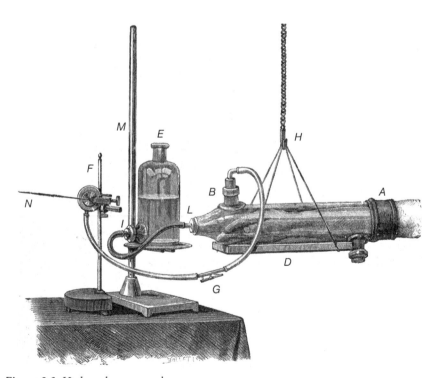

Figure 2.2 Hydrosphygmograph.

The pulse of the lower thigh was recorded with the help of a tin boot constructed according to the same principle as the hydrosphygmograph. The reader may find a depiction of this apparatus and a description of its operation in Chapter 9.

For me, the Marey sphygmograph served only for the purpose of several comparative observations. From the repeated comparisons of the recordings I obtained through both registration methods, I drew the conviction that without my hydrosphygmograph, I would never have succeeded in recognizing the correspondence of the circulatory conditions in the brain with those of other parts of the body, so much do the brain's pulsations deviate in their configuration from the usual depiction of the tracings one obtains of the radial artery with the Marey sphygmograph.

Aside from the threefold problem that with the use of the latter no continuous recording was possible, a reproducibly identical application of the instrument was difficult to achieve, and the pressure was not constant, which makes the Marey instrument unsuitable for prolonged observations and for comparative experiments—I also noticed during my last investigations of the pulse that the Marey sphygmograph distorted the pulsations very considerably due to the resistance of the metallic spring/stylus, which is why one frequently fails to see particulars in the recordings that can be observed in the cerebral pulse and that also appear in the pulse of the forearm as soon as one puts into use the much more sensitive hydrosphygmograph.

The alterations in the volume of the forearm were recorded by means of the plethysmograph described in my treatise *Sopra un nuovo metodo per scrivere I movimenti dei vasi sanguini dell'uomo* (Accademia delle scienze di Torino, novembre 1875). Prof. Cyon has given the necessary instructions for the use of the plethysmograph in his *Methodik* (1876, p. 557).

In order to avoid repetition, I will note once and for all that all tracings provided in the present treatise are inscribed from left to right. With regard to the precision of the woodcuts, I must emphasize that the original data were first reproduced photographically onto wood, whereupon they were carved with all their details and with the greatest precision into the same wood. The tables were initially photographed onto glass according to a new, so-called *photo-zincographic* method and were then etched directly onto zinc by photochemical means, a process that was carried out at the topographic institute of the war ministry in Florence.

NOTES

1. Marey: *Travaux du laboratoire en* 1875, p. 32.
2. Salathé: *Recherches sur les mouvements du cerveau*. Paris, 1877, p. 74.
3. Such glass containers of different sizes are manufactured in the Greiner and Friedrichs factory at Stützerbach. I procured the rubber sleeves from the factory of Pirelli and Casassa in Milan and Turin.

General Considerations Regarding the Configuration of the Pulse

§. 3.1

No part of the body reveals a pulse as variable in its configuration as does the brain. Nonetheless, the most common form of the cerebral pulse, and probably the one to be regarded as normal, is the *tricuspid*. I use this term in its most customary sense, meaning that at the crown of each pulse wave three peaks are noted, of which the middle one is the highest and constitutes the peak of the wave. The deviation of this pulse configuration from the one that since the time of Marey had been considered the norm for the great arterial trunks by all physiologists is so significant that during my first observations, I almost assumed that the brain had a pulse type entirely its own.

However, the investigations I performed to resolve the question of whether there were also other body parts that, under favorable circumstances, could exhibit a pulse configuration analogous to that of the cerebral pulse led to a positive result: They demonstrated in the most definite way that one can obtain at the forearm, the carotid, and the nasal cavity a form of pulsation that corresponds altogether with that of the cerebral pulse. Since the arrangement of the three peaks in the sphygmographic wave contour varies according to different circumstances, I will indicate the means by which I was able to produce these variations at will.

In order not to add to the confusion in this field, I will refrain as much as possible from the introduction of new names and use the designations that have been suggested by the most recent researchers. Thus, we will distinguish, together with Landois, in each wave of the pulse tracing an ascending leg, a peak, and a descending leg, and we will, according to this same researcher's procedure, use the terms *anacrotic* for the elevations perceptible in the ascending wave portion and *catacrotic* for those appearing in the descending portion. Accordingly, we will designate a pulse wave as generally anacrotic when, except for the peak, it shows only anacrotic elevations, and as catacrotic when only the descending leg reveals secondary elevations, and the two, moreover, without regard to the supposed significance of the individual elevations. My tricuspid configuration distinguishes itself from both of the aforementioned pulse waveforms by showing, next to the peak, respective anacrotic and catacrotic elevations.

The terminology of the pulse doctrine becomes more difficult when the issue is to designate the specific individual anacrotic or catacrotic elevations upon which our attention must be directed. Since the designations *dicrotic* and *tricotic* pulse did not suffice for interpretation, Landois assigned to the most substantial of the catacrotic ascents the name *recoil elevation* (*Rückstosselevation*). This appears approximately halfway through the descending wave leg and was formerly called *dicrotic after-beat* (*dicrotischer Nachschlag*). The remaining, more numerous and smaller rises of the pulse wave he called *elasticity elevations*, and in Figure 35 of his *Lehrbuch der Physiologie* (1897, p. 137), these are labeled with the letter *e*. In many of his pulse tracings, he further differentiates a rise situated between the peak and the recoil elevation, which he labels with the letter *k* and which (for reasons that are in my estimation not pertinent) he derives from the closure of the semilunar valves of the aorta (cf. Landois, op. cit., Fig. 35, XI, cited as an example of the pulse of the crural artery). It is incomprehensible to us that he does not make this distinction in other, rather similarly shaped pulse tracings, but instead labels all secondary elevations (except for the recoil elevation) with the letter *e*. For this reason alone, it seems that his special terminology for the individual secondary elevations of the pulse wave is not acceptable.

Furthermore, since the nomenclature suggested by Landois, as per its derivation, involves the concepts of those seminal causal moments postulated by the author, its future fate is tied to the defensibility of Landois's theory. It runs the risk of falling into oblivion if it is not confirmed that the elevation *k* is based on the closure of the semilunar valves, that the so-called recoil elevation rests on a wave motion caused by the rebound thrust of the blood, and that the other elevations are contingent on elasticity.

I believe I am not being too harsh in holding that up until now the origin and the nature of the sphygmic phenomena have not been explained with the degree of precision required in scientific matters. It is my conviction that the experiments we find itemized at length in works on the topic of circulation represent preliminary trials rather than a rigorous analysis of the phenomena noticeable within the pulse wave; I hope not to be blamed if, for cautionary reasons, I reject names that would include a completed interpretation for matters as yet unexplained and insufficiently known.

Since this involves a prominent physiologist like Landois, whose views have found general acceptance in Germany, I will emphasize that I am not the only one to have disputed his theory of the recoil wave. After 1877, the year I first published my treatise,[1] Heynsius and Moens, who studied the matter very thoroughly and successfully, published in 1878 a very interesting work on the pulse configuration,[2] in which they opposed the validity of Landois's theory on the dicrotic elevation. I will go even further and state (and I hope no one will take offense to such an assertion) that Landois's theory of the recoil elevation is incomprehensible to me.

One of the circumstances that caused me great perplexity in the choice of appropriate differential names for the individual elevations of the sphygmographically represented pulse wave was the fact that the normal pulse type, as it results from my observations of the brain and of other body parts, deviates substantially from the model accepted until now as the most usual. This deviation does not hinge on some imperfection of the method I employed for recording the pulse, but rather depends on the greater sensitivity of the same in comparison to the usual sphygmographic methods. The rapidity with which the pulse wave is propagated along the forearm is so great in comparison to the speed of the cylinder's rotation that the tracing of the volume changes of the forearm equals that which we obtain when we record at any one point, by means of a highly sensitive sphygmograph, the pulsations of the walls of the radial artery.

Anacrotism is, in my opinion, a physiologic phenomenon observable under certain circumstances in everyone, without necessitating the presence of the least sign of semilunar valve insufficiency or of aortic aneurysm (to which this phenomenon was generally believed to be linked). By means of various local influences, we can, indeed, render the pulse artificially anacrotic or catacrotic, without cardiac movements undergoing the least modification.

I hope to bring proof that the sphygmic phenomena, with the sole exception of their rhythm and, in part, the height of the pulse, have nothing to do with the heart—that all the remaining characteristic features of the pulse depend solely on the vessels within which, according to the respective condition of the vascular walls of the arterial trunk, the wave of blood projected by the heart undergoes its manifold modifications.

I will endeavor to develop and to justify this view in a subsequent treatise, for which I have already assembled quite a number of experiments that were carried out according to new and precise methods. For now, it may suffice to outline the status of the question. Although in many ways I come close to the ideas expressed recently by Heynsius and Moens on the nature of dicrotism, I reserve the right in my future work on the nature of sphygmic phenomena to take various exceptions to the views of these researchers.

It is their opinion that the dicrotic elevation does not stem from a reflection but simply from the closure of the semilunar valve, which is why they suggest the term *closing wave*. While I admire the precision with which Heynsius and Moens carried out their investigations and willingly recognize their merit in having provided a fresh impetus to the study of the pulse, I must nevertheless confess that I would not have dared to draw too many conclusions from the phenomena they observed during the opening and closing of two containers connected by an elastic tube. I suspect that (1) the walls of the tube used for their observations were much too distensible in comparison to those of the aorta and of other arteries; (2) the levels of pressure employed were too low; and (3) the two wave factors (i.e., the opening and closing of the spigot that substituted for the aortic cusps) were temporally too far apart.

It is for these reasons that I consider it requisite, if only as a precaution, to reject, for the time being, the appellation *closing wave* to designate the dicrotic elevation. I will hold fast to the old designations as long as Heynsius and Moens's theory is not confirmed by new and more convincing experiments. The term *dicrotic elevation*, aside from its right of priority, also has the advantage that it does not include any preconception as to the cause of the phenomenon and thus leaves an open field for discussion.

As for the previously mentioned rise located between the primary and the dicrotic elevation, which Landois at times designates with the letter *k* and attributes to the closure of the aortic valve cusps, Heynsius has introduced the term *elevation S* and believes that, on the contrary, this rise represents the manifestation of a wave movement *effecting* the valve closure. We will, in honor of Heynsius, accept his designation all the more willingly since it merits, simply because of its consequential execution, pre-eminence over that of Landois.

In addition, I am also of the opinion that the elevation in question cannot, as Landois assumes, stem from the closure of the aortic cusps, for in the course of a series of investigations on the relationships between the heart sounds and rises of the pulse wave I did not find any constant relationship between the two series of phenomena. It is true that this negative result would also be in opposition to Heynsius's theory. However, I dare not speak out definitively as to this question, since the method I have used until now to resolve it has been inadequate.

§. 3.2

The tricuspid pulse is not exclusive to the brain because I have often encountered it in the forearm, in the carotid, and in the great intrathoracic vessels.

These, as well as other pulse configurations, are manifestations that depend on the condition of the vessels. Indeed, as soon as a contraction of the vascular walls occurs, for instance, we notice that the earlier tricuspid or anacrotic pulse of an artery or an organ becomes catacrotic.

Here is an example of the successive variations in contour that the cerebral pulse undergoes as a result of the contraction of the cerebral blood vessels, shown in Fig. 3.1.

Bertino remained perfectly still. His brain had experienced, due to a preceding stimulus, a significant expansion in volume, and its pulsations, which can be seen at the onset of the tracing in Fig. 3.1, had become very high and tricuspid.

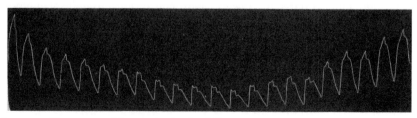

Figure 3.1 Variations of the cerebral pulse following a contraction of the cerebral vessels.

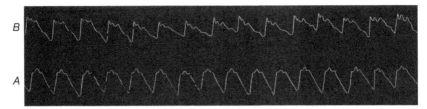

Figure 3.2 *A:* Forearm pulse in the setting of perfect mental repose. *B:* Forearm pulse of the same person with increased mental activity.

Suddenly, and without any cause known to me, the undulation visible in the subsequent tracing of the same pulse wave set in; volume diminished, and the pulse became catacrotic.

Such phenomena occurred repeatedly, in my observations of Bertino as well as of Catherina X. and of Thron, and I would not know how to explain these other than by the assumption of a vascular contraction, as I will clarify in Chapter 7.

The pulse in the forearm can take the same shape as that in the brain and can present the same spontaneous transformations, as can be seen in the tracing in Fig. 3.2. Wave *A* represents the forearm pulse of Mr. Caudana in the horizontal position and at complete rest. The upper wave *B* was recorded a minute later, while I spoke to Mr. Caudana.

In order to determine the extent of vascular contraction during such variations of the pulse wave, I measured the degree of volume diminution in Dr. Cervello through simultaneous use of the plethysmograph and the hydrosphygmograph (see Fig. 3.3).

We see that while his resting pulse was tricuspid, as in tracing *A*, it became strongly catacrotic following the inhalation of ammonia. The pulsations, which in tracing *A* show a catacrotic shape, coincide with inspiration. In the subsequent minute, while the volume of the forearm diminished by 16 cm^3, the pulse had the configuration represented in tracing *B*.

The contraction of the vessels continued further so that in the course of a minute I observed a decrease in volume of over 20 cm^3.

This experiment is also of interest from a pharmacologic standpoint. I have carried it out over the course of several years during my lectures on pharmacology in order to demonstrate the influence of ammonia upon the blood vessels and to show the mode of action of this substance in its most usual medical

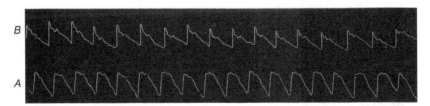

Figure 3.3 *A:* Forearm pulse in the normal state. *B:* Its change after inhalation of ammonia.

application. A medication that in such a short period of time can cause the passage (efflux) of more than 20 cm³ of blood from only one forearm to the inner body parts can understandably provide a valuable service when the goal is to propel blood from the periphery to the central organs, in order to stimulate the circulation and to restore the functions of the nerve centers.

§. 3.3

Mental activity is also one of the means by which one can easily transform the tricuspid pulse into a catacrotic one. To demonstrate this, it suffices to wait until the person who is the subject of our experiment is at complete rest and then to ask him any discretionary question, inviting him, for instance, to solve an arithmetic task (Fig. 3.4).

Fig. 3.4 is a hydrosphygmographic tracing of the forearm pulse of medical student Mr. Riva. The pulse is tripartite. At point ⇓ I invited the gentleman to multiply 22 by 14. An initial, slight volume decrease of the forearm ensued. Thereafter, the pulse became smaller and more frequent, while the volume underwent a transient increase. Then a more substantial decrease in volume took place, during which the frequency of the heartbeats was slightly diminished. The profile of the tracing became catacrotic.

When the elevation S is not visible in the forearm pulse, it is enough to cause a contraction of the vessels in order for that elevation to appear. Fig. 3.5 shows an example of such a transformation of the pulse induced by mental activity.

I found in the same medical student, Mr. Riva, that the forearm pulse was catacrotic with deep rest (tracing A). At point ⇓ (tracing B), I asked the gentleman to multiply 171 by 5. The vascular contraction effected during this intensified intellectual activity was accompanied by the intensification of elevation S, which was not noticeable beforehand. I made sure that the lack of this elevation in tracing A was not due to excessive pressure of the stylus upon the rotating cylinder.

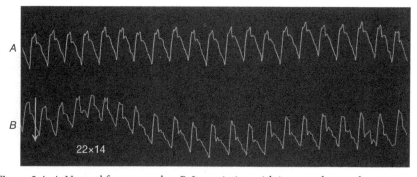

Figure 3.4 *A:* Normal forearm pulse. *B:* Its variation with increased mental activity.

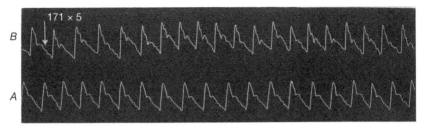

Figure 3.5 Appearance of the elevation *S* in pulse tracing *B* following increased mental activity.

In the chapter on sleep, we will see that one of the conditions necessary for the tricuspid form to be manifest as the normal, typical configuration of the pulse consists of deep repose of the person subjected to observation. As soon as the psychic centers enter into intensified activity, or as the transition from sleep to the waking state takes place, the profile of the pulsations in the brain as well as in the forearm changes immediately; conversely, the tricuspid shape is resumed when we return to the earlier resting state.

§. 3.4

In my study on the diagnosis of the pulse,[3] a special chapter is devoted to the **"Configuration of the pulse with an empty stomach and after the intake of food."** Here the contrast is generally so great that one can easily distinguish even with a cursory glance the tracings obtained in the fasting state from those taken after a meal. To give an example of the great ease with which the eye recognizes the characteristic signs of the pulse, I will mention that during cursory leafing through my collection of original sphygmographic tables I can distinguish right away, without reading any marginal notes or reviewing the diary, the sphygmograms taken in the morning and in the afternoon, after breakfast or after lunch.

I am not referring here to the variety of rhythm, for it was known long ago that the heart contracts faster after meals than before meals. Our attention must instead be directed exclusively to the contour of the pulse and must be restricted to the consideration of the manner in which the three previously mentioned elevations are arranged. With a few exceptions, one may accept as a rule that the shape of the pulse is **tricuspid in the fasting state** and that it **becomes catacrotic after a meal** (Fig. 3.6).

Of the numerous examples I could cite in support of this phenomenon, I choose two tracings, which I recorded using Dr. Pagliani and Dr. Albertotti on a day that I had invited them to breakfast with me in my laboratory. They had fasted until 1 PM. I need hardly note that I had taken every precaution to eliminate any potential source of error originating from a different method of application of the hydrosphygmograph.

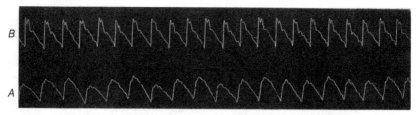

Figure 3.6 *A:* Forearm pulse of Prof. Pagliani in the fasting state. *B:* Id. after breakfast.

On the same occasion, my own pulse was also recorded before and after break-fast. A simple examination of these tracings is enough to convince oneself that there exists a fundamental difference between pulse waves before and after a meal. A large intake of food into our body is enough to change the configuration of the pulse after absorption of soluble or digestible substances and to make it catacrotic (Fig. 3.7).

Elsewhere, I have already expressed my conviction that the main reason for this change resides in the increase of the tone of the vascular walls (Fig 3.8).

In fact, this view is confirmed by the analogy that forces us to compare the present phenomenon to others, where the appearance of a vascular contraction is demonstrated in the most unquestionable way. I hope that I will soon be able to furnish other, even more convincing evidence for this, which will be drawn from my series of investigations started long ago about the elasticity of the vascular walls.

As regards the changes undergone by the cerebral pulse under the influence of nutritional intake, I have only one observation, which I made of Bertino on the day he visited me in my laboratory. After recording six pages with the Marey cylinder, we rested for 1 hour. The last tracings obtained with an empty stomach are noted in the next chapter (on increased mental activity). As soon as noon struck, I interrupted our session; freed Bertino's arm from the plethysmograph after having marked it with ink on the skin of the elbow, the site where the rubber sleeve was located; and left in place on Bertino's head the gutta percha plate. I then invited the man to have lunch with me, and he took a copious amount of bread, sausage, cheese, fruit, and two glasses of white Cannelli wine. At 1 PM I resumed observation, having carefully restored the earlier conditions, and

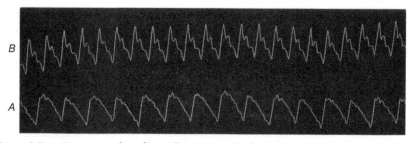

Figure 3.7 *A:* Forearm pulse of Dr. Albertotti in the fasting state. *B:* Id. after breakfast.

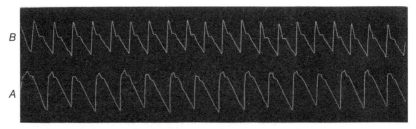

Figure 3.8 *A:* My forearm pulse in the fasting state. *B:* Id. after breakfast.

recorded four more pages. On these tracings (of which in Plate 4.1, 5, *AC*, I reproduce only one that consists of approximately 1 minute and was obtained about 1 and a half hours after the meal), one can clearly recognize that the cerebral pulse has also turned catacrotic. In doing so, it has become smaller and much more regular.

§. 3.5

I stated previously that the tricuspid pulse is a manifestation dependent on the condition of the blood vessels. I will now offer the evidence for this assertion.

If we simultaneously trace the cerebral and the carotid pulses, we find very frequently that the first is tricuspid while the other appears catacrotic (Fig. 3.9).

The tracing at hand demonstrates that the wave of blood, during transition from the carotid trunk to its branchings, has become tricuspid.

In the same way, if we simultaneously record the carotid pulse and that of the forearm, we can satisfy ourselves that the tripartite pulse represents a peripheral phenomenon, in that the pulsations are catacrotic in the carotid whereas in the forearm they appear as tricuspid.

A further and even more compelling argument for the independence of this pulse wave from the heart is brought by the fact that also under normal circumstances, the pulse can be anacrotic in one forearm and catacrotic in the other. Of

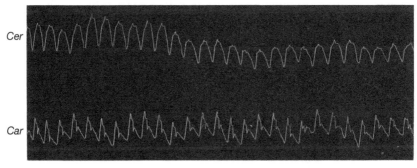

Figure 3.9 Carotid pulse *Car*, recorded at the same time as the cerebral pulse *Cer*.

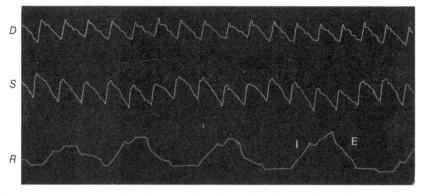

Figure 3.10 Pulse of the right forearm *D* and of the left *S*, recorded at the same time as respiration *R*.

the numerous examples I could cite, the present one may serve as evidence for my statement (Fig. 3.10).

The superior tracing *D* pertains to the right forearm, the second *S* to the left; the third *R* represents respiration, recorded simultaneously by means of the Marey cardiograph. I need hardly stress that I would not have thought this finding decisive if I had not assured myself that the difference between both forearms remained the same when I exchanged their respective recording tambours. The tracing *R* rises during inspiration and falls during expiration, as the annotated letters *I* and *E* indicate. The volume of the left forearm reveals fluctuations that correspond to the respiratory phases. We will discuss this phenomenon at greater length in Chapters 9 to 11; at present it should suffices for us to note that the pulse is modified by respiratory movements. The most distinctly tricuspid pulsations of the tracing under consideration correspond to the end of expiration, and the exquisitely catacrotic ones to the end of inspiration.

Everyone will easily understand that such observations incited my desire to determine more exactly the circumstances of this phenomenon, and that my entire attention had to be directed to the search for the most expedient process for making the pulse of one forearm anacrotic and unchanged in the other. I could not think of any other way to arrive at an understanding of the basis for such a transformation in the shape of the pulse.

One of the first methods I found suitable for making the pulse tricuspid in one forearm and at the same time keeping it catacrotic in the other consists of introducing each forearm initially into a hydrosphygmograph and comparing the pulse reaction in both extremities at the normal ambient temperature (34°C); thereafter, the forearm is cooled inside the hydrosphygmograph in question by filling the glass cylinder with water at 6°C or 7°C, and then it is gradually warmed by the introduction of increasingly warmer water into the glass cylinder, until the temperature has reached 40°C to 42°C. As a consequence of this variation in temperature, the vessels expand in a quite extraordinary fashion, and the

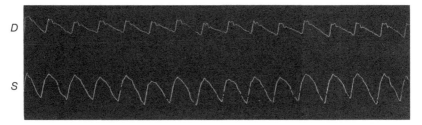

Figure 3.11 Variation of the left forearm pulse *S* under the influence of temperature, while on the right side the pulse *D* remains normal.

higher their degree of immobilization, the more distinct the appearance of the tricuspid pulse form (Fig. 3.11).

I tried an experiment on myself. I applied a hydrosphygmograph to each forearm and first ascertained that the pulse of both extremities was nearly equal in nature. Then I cooled the water in the left glass cylinder down to 7°C and subsequently heated it quickly to 36°C. Tracing *S* in Fig. 3.11 represents the pulse of the left forearm, tracing *D* that of the right. In the first the pulse appears as tricuspid; in the other it appears as catacrotic.

Another, even simpler way to transform the catacrotic pulse of only one forearm into an anacrotic one consists of a prolonged muscular contraction, whether such may happen voluntarily or be provoked by means of the induction current. To this matter I have already devoted an entire chapter in my work on the local variations of the pulse, and I will cite here only two examples to demonstrate that in this manner the forearm pulse can be made entirely equal to that of the brain, as is seen in the tracings in Fig. 3.12, obtained on Mr. Roth. Tracing *A* in Fig. 3.12 represents the pulse of the right forearm in the normal state, tracing *B* the pulse of the same extremity approximately 10 minutes after the end of a contraction provoked by an induction current lasting 40 seconds.

The catacrotic right forearm pulse of the same Mr. Roth, represented here by tracing *A* in Fig. 3.13, was transformed into a tricuspid one (tracing *B*) after a voluntary, tonic muscle contraction (forceful clenching of the fist) had taken place, and indeed after having lasted barely 30 seconds.

The change in the pulse wave is much more difficult to elicit in the great vascular trunks, and the previously mentioned methods are only valid for the total pulse (volume fluctuations) of the body parts.

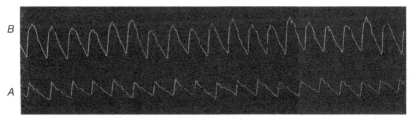

Figure 3.12 *A:* Normal forearm pulse. *B:* Variation of the latter following a muscular contraction caused by induction current.

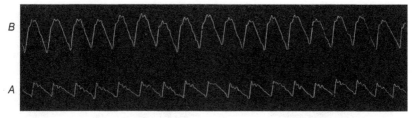

Figure 3.13 *A:* Normal forearm pulse. *B:* Variation of the latter following a voluntary muscle contraction.

The experiments discussed (as can be observed in the results obtained) were collectively aimed at lowering, by as high a degree as possible, the tone of the arterial walls in the branches of an arterial trunk. Using amyl nitrite, I succeeded in a few cases to bring about such an extensive paralysis of the vessels that even in the carotid the pulse became anacrotic, as can be seen in the recording in Fig. 3.14 tracing *A*, obtained on Mr. Garzena. Due to space constraints I only reproduce a fragment of the pair of tracings obtained, that is, a portion that was registered approximately 8 seconds after the end of the amyl nitrite inhalation. In the first few pulsations, the anacrotism can still be recognized; this dissipates later on, to the extent that the effect of amyl nitrite wears off. A similar transformation reveals itself in the forearm, where the pulse was recorded simultaneously (tracing *A*). We see indeed, to the extent that the normal condition is re-established, the dicrotic increase approach the peak of the wave ever more closely.

The increase *S* can be made to disappear through simple pressure on the surface of the vessels. In fact, after I observed this rise in the pulse of Mr. Garzena, I attached a tube to the cylindrical glass container by means of which, after filling it with water, I exerted a pressure of approximately 20 cm (ca. 15 mm of mercury) onto the forearm and then continued to record its volume changes in the same manner. The increase *S* disappeared, while the dicrotic and tricrotic rises became much more pronounced (Fig. 3.15).

The first pulse increase *S* is at times so faintly indicated that it barely produces a slight, wavy curvature of the ascending leg of the pulse wave, which thereby acquires, instead of a linear shape as was already pointed out by Landois,[4] a very elongated, S-shaped contour.

If we produce an increase in cerebral volume by preventing the outflow of blood, as happens with compression of the jugular veins, then this increase is immediately apparent in the ascending leg of the wave, and the previously

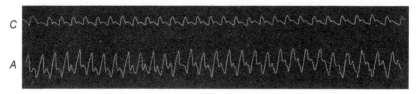

Figure 3.14 Carotid pulse *C* and forearm pulse *A* during inhalation of amyl nitrite.

catacrotic pulse becomes anacrotic. The reader will find examples of such variations of the cerebral pulse in Chapter 13 on the hyperemia and anemia of the
brain.

The Marey sphygmograph could not generate the increase S as a constant factor of the sphygmographic tracing, because the pressure of the stylus distorts
the recording and augments the dicrotism in the same way as with the use of
the hydrosphygmograph, as soon as we raise the pressure above the usual level.

Nevertheless, even though it is more sensitive than the Marey sphygmograph,
the hydrosphygmograph, too, presents certain obstacles to the depiction of the
three characteristic elevations in the first half of the pulse wave. If the peak of the
wave is rounded, it is often possible to discern the elevation S with a magnifying
glass; alternatively, one can bring it forth by lessening the pressure of the writing
stylus upon the coated paper of the kymograph cylinder, as well as by diminish-
ing the friction through a weaker coating of the paper.

I will first expand the field of my observations before discussing the mechanical conditions that are the basis for the anacrotism of the pulse. However,
what I have written on this topic in the present chapter will hopefully suffice
to stimulate a more precise investigation of a phenomenon that until now has
been regarded as pertaining exclusively to the field of pathology (Landois, op.
cit. p. 254), yet which we must focus on as a normal manifestation of the pulse of
various organs.

Since Landois was the first to conduct, by schematic means, inquiries into the
causes that might lie at the root of the anacrotic increases, I consider it my duty
to conclude this chapter by citing his words[5] in which he summarizes the general
conditions for the origination of the anacrotic pulse:

> In very general terms, the anacrotism will take place when the time period
> within which the elastic tube experiences the highest degree of expansion, is
> longer than the number of oscillations (*Schwingungszahl*) of the extended/
> tightened tubal wall. Thus, all factors, which prolong the time to maximal
> expansion, or increase the number of oscillations of the extended elastic
> wall, will be capable of causing anacrotic elevations. However, the amount
> of time within which the elastic tube experiences the highest degree of
> expansion depends on the force of the pressure with which the quantity of

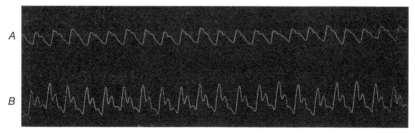

Figure 3.15 Transformation of the forearm pulse *A* into *B* through the pressure of a
column of water measuring 20 cm.

fluid is propelled into the elastic tube. Those are the moments on which the appearance of anacrotic elevations can be dependent.

NOTES

1. A. Mosso: *Die Diagnostik des Pulses.* Leipzig, 1879.
2. Dr. A. Isebree Moens: *Die Pulscurve.* Leiden, 1878.
3. A. Mosso: *Die Diagnostik des Pulses.* Leipzig, 1879, p. 14.
4. Landois: *Die Lehre vom Arterienpulse.* Berlin, 1872, p. 151.
5. Ibid.

Concerning the Response of the Cerebral Circulation During Increased Mental Activity and With Emotional and Sensory Perceptions

§. 4.1

The study of the modifications the blood circulation undergoes under the influence of psychic activity can be extraordinarily difficult if one wants to separate the variations of blood flow limited solely to the brain from those that involve the entire vascular system and that are based on the fluctuations of the strength and rate of the cardiac contractions, or on general variations of blood pressure.

Since the brain belongs to the organs removed from direct voluntary control, and since we are nominally in the position to force it at will to an absolute state of rest, the changes that its blood flow can undergo in the waking state are contingent much more often upon fluctuations in the vigorousness of the mental activity than on a true transition of the psychic centers from a state of absolute rest to one of full activity.

In this instance, we will first cite an experiment performed with Bertino on September 23, 1878.

Plate 4.1 (p. 61) depicts the successive changes the pulse undergoes simultaneously in the brain (C) and in the forearm (A) over the course of 5 minutes.

Bertino's pulse was traced for approximately 1½ hours. The right forearm was enclosed within the hydrosphygmograph, and on the skull defect was placed the gutta percha plate through which the cranial cavity was connected to the recording barrel.

Early in the morning, Bertino ate a *minestra*.[1] He was in a state of complete rest and was distracted.

The two lines of tracings that were registered before tracing 1 *AC* and that I omitted to save space are almost perfectly horizontal; only now and then does the brain show slight, elongated undulations that are similar to tracing 1 *C*.

In the first half of the forearm tracing 1 *A*, we notice two rather substantial oscillations *m* and *n*, which are probably due to deeper respiratory movements. Because my attention was occupied by something else at that moment, I missed the change that had taken place in the forearm pulse. I only noticed it at the subsequent rotation of the cylinder, and fearing that it might have stemmed from a hand movement, I asked Bertino to remain totally immobile. This request, which I addressed to him at the beginning of lines 2 *AC*, he interpreted as a reproach, because I had pressed him several times earlier to remain absolutely still. As a result of the mood swing induced by this thought, we see that the cerebral pulse in the tracing lines 2 *AC* turns out to be somewhat higher than before. At point *a* I asked the man whether he was thinking about something specific. He responded "no"; nonetheless, I believe that his emotional state had been manifestly agitated by my words.

During the tracing of lines 3 *AC*, both of us remained silent. At the onset of these lines there are three or four more rapid heartbeats, and immediately thereafter a few more sporadic/slower ones. The respective cerebral and forearm volumes responded in a completely different way during this variation of the cardiac rhythm; indeed, while the pulsations of the forearm (line *A*) fell, those of the brain (line *C*) rose. I believe the changed rhythm of the heartbeats alone was not sufficient to cause this inverse relationship, but that at the same time a contraction of the forearm vessels had to have taken place, which resulted in a further volume increase of the brain. In the second half of the tracing 3 *AC*, the cerebral pulse increased again in amplitude without the operation of a known stimulus or the presence of a visible change of the forearm pulse. Later on (in the continuation, not reproduced here, of the said tracing), the cerebral pulse wave fell anew and returned to its original height.

At the start of lines 4 *AC*, a colleague entered the room and began to look attentively at Bertino and at the apparatus in operation. The height of the cerebral pulsations and the volume of the brain—and thus the flow of blood to this organ—increased significantly. Toward the middle of the tracing Bertino spontaneously moved his finger, as can be discerned in the deviation *p*, which appears in the middle of line *A*. Thereafter followed a 5-minute pause.

§. 4.2

After my colleague left and I saw that Bertino had again become quite still, I recorded the lines 1 *AC* of Fig. 4.1, in which one can see that the cerebral and forearm pulses have regained their normal shape. In the next minute, I asked Bertino how many eggs there are in two dozens.

The earlier experiments had taught me that in order to sustain his attention, it was necessary to formulate a question (for instance, a multiplication task) as a more concrete problem he might encounter in his day-to-day life as a peasant. Multiplying abstract numbers seemed to him but an idle game, and thus he did not consider this with the same vivid interest.

Unfortunately, the man moved his fingers, and the forearm tracing was disfigured as a result. Because of this, I scolded him in a rather strong tone of voice. But since I had given him a similar reprimand half an hour earlier, he was somewhat offended by my words; I noticed at the beginning of the subsequently recorded pair of tracings that his face had reddened more intensely and that he kept his eyes fixed on the ground with embarrassment.

I omit the pair of lines in question and reproduce the tracing 2 *AC* obtained 30 minutes later, at a time when the consequences of emotional agitation are still very visible.

The cerebral pulsations are higher; one notices a concomitant change of those of the forearm. The rate of cardiac contractions remains almost constant.

In the paired tracings 2 *AC*, where the ⇓ is noted, the pendulum clock in the room struck 12, and at the same time one heard the bell of the neighboring church. The unexpected impact of this sound was followed by a marked change of brain volume and by a greater amplitude of the pulsations.

If I had reproduced in Fig. 4.1 the direct continuation of lines 2 *AC*, one would notice in it a very high degree of increase in blood flow to the brain: The 20th pulsation of line *C* following the symbol ⇓ (which corresponds to the first peal of the clock striking noon) went so far beyond the upper line *A* of the forearm pulsations that I was forced to vent the release valve (clarinet) in order to prevent excessive tension of the tambour membrane.

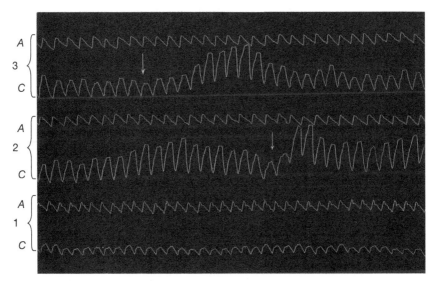

Figure 4.1 Changes of the cerebral blood circulation under the influence of mental processes. Forearm pulse *A* and cerebral pulse *C*, recorded simultaneously.

I need hardly remark that in the course of these experiments to determine the relationships between cerebral activity and blood circulation, I made use of all precautions necessary to ensure the reliability of the results. The room was chosen because of its complete isolation, so that no exterior noise could be heard; moreover, I had asked Dr. De Paoli to stand behind the patient's back. The most stringent provision, to which I, too, subjected myself, was not to move and not to speak except in the case of absolute necessity. Bertino sat facing the wall, so that he would not perceive any intercurrent facial expressions except for those I wanted him to see.

After a minute the clock struck 12 for the second time. This repetition of the sound produced a less striking effect in the cerebral circulation. (The tracing in question is not reproduced.)

Since I had been struck by the extraordinary increase of the cerebral pulsation after the ringing of the church bells had begun, especially since at the same time the radial pulse had only undergone a relatively minimal modification, I asked Bertino at point ⇓ of line 3 *AC* (i.e., about 1 minute after the second striking of the clock) whether he was in the habit of reciting the Ave Maria at noontime. This question occurred to me because of my suspicion that the important change in the cerebral circulation when the clock struck 12 was possibly related to the emotion that manifested itself in the man because at noontime he could not, as is the custom of our rural people, make the sign of the cross or say a prayer. In fact, Bertino answered that he did at times recite the Ave Maria.

Having noted this increase in cerebral volume and pulse amplitude under the influence of mental activity and of sensory and emotional perceptions, we will endeavor to analyze these phenomena more closely and to determine their cause and their mechanism.

Let us consider another tracing of Bertino's mental activity, where during the intellectual operation there was no accidental movement of the fingers on his part to interfere in a disruptive way, as occurred during the recording of one of the tracings in Fig. 4.1.

If we observe the pulse tracings of the brain and of the forearm in Plate 4.1, line pairs 5 *AC*, we notice immediately that here they show a different profile from that of the previous experiment. However, here the type of the pulsations is different for the simple reason that Bertino had been fasting during the recording, whereas the tracing that presently concerns us was obtained after he had already lunched.

We will return to this matter later on, in Chapter 11. For now, it is enough for me to draw attention to the fact that as a result of nutritional intake into the organism, both the pulse of Bertino's brain as well as that of his forearm had undergone a significant change.

At the point of insertion of the symbol ⇓ in Plate 4.1, line pairs 5 *AC*, I asked the man to multiply 8 times 22. At point *ω* Bertino told me the obtained product. We see that the cerebral pulse remained increased during the entire duration of the arithmetic operation; Fig. 4.2 shows us another example of the modifications the cerebral blood circulation undergoes in the course of a mental task. Where

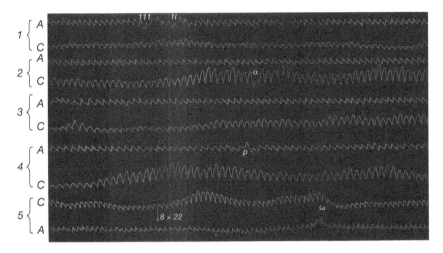

Plate 4.1

the symbol $\mu \Downarrow$ is located, I had Bertino multiply 8 by 12. Here, too, one clearly sees that the amplitude of the pulsations and the cerebral volume increase at the start of the mental task.

From these tracings one learns furthermore that the variation of the blood flow is more marked at the start and at the end of the mental task; indeed, at times it is only noticeable at all at the start and at the end. In fact, psychic performance/activity is most intense at the moment when the task is taken up, as well as at the moment when its result is pronounced.

As to what happens during mental activity in the vasculature of other body parts, I have already shown this in two other works where I first demonstrated the volume changes of the forearm[2] following a simple multiplication and the subsequently generated transformations of the forearm pulse.[3] Those two series of experiments have demonstrated that during mental activity there is a strong vascular contraction that takes place in the forearm.[4]

My results of those early investigations were confirmed later on by other researchers, among whom I especially note Prof. Thanhoffer, who has recently published a series of related data.[5]

It is probable that the contraction noticed in the vessels of both arms also takes place in the lower extremities and in the entire exterior skin of the body. In any case, however, when blood vessels in a certain state of expansion contract in the

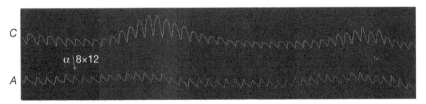

Figure 4.2 Cerebral pulse C and forearm pulse A, recorded at the same time as an enhanced mental activity.

course of more intense cerebral activity, because of the increase in pressure a passive expansion must take place in other vascular regions.

According to the experiments of Thanhoffer, the latter phenomenon occurs even in the larger and medium-size arteries of the same extremities, in which we demonstrated a change in volume, that is, an obvious narrowing of the smallest vessels. In fact, he found (upon application of the Marey sphygmograph to the radial artery) a *widening* of this vessel with increased mental activity. The general increase of blood pressure in the vascular system brought about by a local contraction of the vascular walls must indeed lead to a widening of the vascular lumen in those vessel regions or portions where the *muscularis* either is weak or does not participate in the ongoing contraction. And it is this mechanism that, in our case, is responsible for the vascular expansion in the area of the cerebral arteries and the augmented blood flow to the brain, as well as the widening of the radial artery in Thanhoffer's experiment.

Added to these factors, moreover, is a slight increase in the rate and force of the cardiac contractions.

To put into sharper focus the influence of the heart onto the circulatory manifestations that one observes with greater mental activity, I have provided on page 48, Fig. 3.4, a pulse tracing that reveals that in some individuals, at first, the phenomena that predominate are those that depend on the increased rate of the heartbeats, which is why initially one observes also in the forearm a transient slight increase in volume, followed by a more marked decrease of the forearm volume caused by the contraction of the forearm vessels, which itself is the determining factor.

§. 4.3

As early as 1876, after I had published my first plethysmographic observations on the movements of the blood vessels taking place as a consequence of emotional feelings and of increased intellectual activity, my honored friend Prof. Franck raised the objection that these circulatory changes might be related to an alteration of the respiratory movements.[6] I promised him (in my treatise on the local variations of the pulse) a categorical response, and now I want to keep my promise.

That the changes in forearm volume and the concomitantly noticed increase in brain volume are not related to a modification of the respiratory movements is evidenced by the following circumstances:

1. If we record the forearm pulse and the respiratory movements simultaneously, we find not infrequently that the volume of the forearm diminishes with increased mental activity, while the rhythm and the depth of the respiratory movements remain unchanged.
2. If we record the respiratory graph and the cerebral movements simultaneously, we find that the volume of the brain increases with

more intense mental activity, while the respiratory movements do not experience any changes.

3. The character of the sphygmographic tracing of the forearm reveals that a contraction of the vessels is truly present, and it does not conform to that which the tracing presents with mere modification of the respiratory movements.

4. Since the arteries going to the head and to the upper extremities have a common origin and have the same relationships to the thorax, if the phenomena I attribute to vascular action were really dependent on a change of respiratory movements resulting from increased mental activity, then it is certain that very similar modifications of the pulse would have to occur in both parts of the body (head and arms)—which, however, is not the case. The validity of this argument is all the more obvious when one considers that with increased mental activity we indeed observe the exact opposite, for the volume variation in both body parts takes place in opposite directions—in the head as an increase in cerebral volume and in the upper extremities as a decrease in volume of both forearms—even though the influence of the respiratory movements on the head and the upper limbs is quite identical.

If one investigates in several persons the behavior of the respiratory movements in their relationship to mental activity, it becomes impossible to reduce the perceived variations to a single type.

The pertinent observations, which I had already undertaken in 1874 (when I was working in Ludwig's laboratory), have up until now not furnished any satisfactory results—so manifold were the respiratory types that I found in a great number of individuals in the setting of continued mental activity.

This extraordinary variability of respiratory movements, compared to the constancy with which, in the presence of increased mental activity, the contraction of the forearm vessels and the augmentation of cerebral volume manifest themselves (as I have confirmed every time on Bertino, as well as on Catherina X. and on Thron), also demonstrates, and exceedingly so, that the respiratory movements cannot be regarded as a causative factor among the phenomena that occupy us in this chapter.

Here, however, we have two examples that reveal that during cerebral activity the brain volume increases without a concomitant change in the rhythm of breathing.

In graph 7, Plate 4.2, the tracing R represents the thoracic respiratory movements recorded at the same time as the cerebral pulse C. Even though the second inspiration is deeper than the first, it has almost no influence on the contour of the cerebral pulse. However, when I asked Bertino to multiply 9 by 13, there was a significant change of the pulse tracing together with an increase in cerebral volume, which ensues without a corresponding change in respiration. In P, Bertino stated the product. Even though at this moment he took a deeper breath than all previous ones, the change of the pulse curve was relatively minimal.

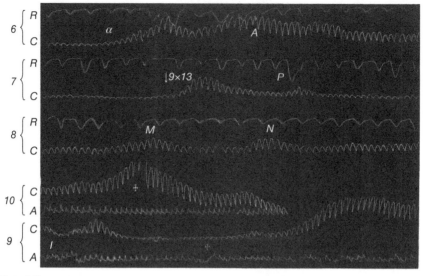

Plate 4.2

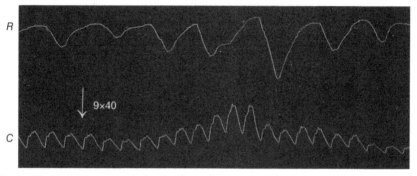

Figure 4.3 The increase in cerebral volume during an intellectual task does not correspond to any change in respiration. *C:* Cerebral pulse. *R:* Respiratory movements of the thorax, traced with a Marey pneumograph.

Fig. 4.3 similarly shows that the variation of the cerebral pulse during mental activity does not at all depend on the variations of respiratory movements. Indeed, when I asked Bertino to multiply 9 by 40, there was an increase in the amplitude of cerebral pulsations, while the more ample respiratory movements only began when the increase in cerebral volume had already taken place.

§. 4.4

In my first study **on the local variations of the pulse,** I had already stated as a general rule that the excitement taking place during the transition from deep rest to mental activity is always accompanied by a modification of the pulse;

however, I had also added that this law did not exclude the possibility that during a protracted and strenuous intellectual task one might not observe any change of the pulse.

The just-mentioned law, as well as its restriction, is also valid for the pulsations of the brain. When Bertino was not in a state of complete rest and his attention not already captured by something, the influence of the transition of the mind to another intellectual task was less obvious in the features of the cerebral blood circulation, and at times not noticeable at all.

The research of pulse fluctuations in the brain is much more difficult than that in the forearm, because even at maximal rest the blood flow within the skull is not evenly maintained. The brain, as I emphasized at the beginning of this chapter, is an organ that eludes our voluntary control; it can be all the more powerfully active the more we want to compel it to relax, and its blood flow can undergo changes even when we are unaware of the organ's activity as is evidenced in Plate 4.2, line pair 8 *RC*.

Bertino was in a profound state of repose. One sees this because of his very regular and flat breathing. In *M* and in *N* we notice an increase in brain volume, in conjunction with an increase in amplitude of the pulsations. However, Bertino had not moved; everything around him had remained still, and I was unable to discover what had affected him. After the recording of the graph lines was complete, I questioned him and he answered that he had not thought about anything and had been very distracted.

As a rule, states of emotional excitement affect the cerebral blood circulation far more conspicuously than does intellectual activity, no matter how energetic it might be. I stated earlier that in the experiment to which the first tracing pertains, I reprimanded Bertino after the end of his multiplication because he had moved his fingers and thereby spoiled the experiment. If we examine the pulsations more carefully, we recognize that they increased after the multiplication had ended.

Among the many examples I could cite as evidence for this fact, I choose one in which the phenomenon stands out in a particularly characteristic way: Plate 4.2, line pairs 9 and 10 *AC*.

At the start of line pair 9, mark *I*, I nodded to Bertino to take two deep inspirations. After he had done so and while I was preoccupied with observing the resulting effects on the forearm and brain, I noticed that he moved his fingers: mark +. I turned to him and told him in a fairly harsh tone of voice: "You behave like a child; you spoil everything for me." Immediately thereafter the cerebral volume increased and the cerebral pulsations became so tall that I had to activate the relief valve twice in order to bring the pressure of the barrel down to zero, the first time at the end of the graph lines, the second time in the upper lines 10 *CA*, where the symbol + is noted. After this mark, the brain volume diminished again and the pulsations gradually returned to their original form, which I could discern in a third pair of lines, which because of space constraints I do not reproduce.

Another time (Plate 4.3, line pairs 11 and 12) when Bertino, in spite of repeated admonitions, had also involuntarily moved a finger (see start of line 11 *A*), I only looked at him angrily; however, he became aware of his carelessness right away, and immediately a widening of the cerebral vessels appeared and at the same time the cerebral pulsations grew to be three to four times higher than before and the brain volume increased markedly, without there having been a detectable change in the forearm. The tracing 12 *AC*, which was obtained right afterward, represents the behavior of the blood flow in the forearm and in the brain in the state of mental repose. At *M* I slightly lifted the styli by means of the static lever, so as not to mar line 11 *C*.

From these examples, as well as from repeated additional observations, it appears that, just as we saw earlier regarding the influence of intellectual effort, the influence of emotions is expressed much less in the circulatory conditions of the forearm than in those of the brain, and, moreover, where it becomes detectable, it manifests itself not through a dilatation, as in the brain, but instead through a narrowing of the vessels. I have already spoken elsewhere of the alterations that the volume of the forearm undergoes under similar conditions; I will therefore restrict myself to one example regarding the pulse contour (Plate 4.3, tracing 13).

At around 10 AM the student Mr. Bosio sat with his forearm in the hydrosphygmograph and kept very still. I had been recording his pulse tracing for about 20 minutes to determine first any potential spontaneous movements of the forearm vessels before moving on to the experiment, which was to consist of the administration of a dose of ergotin. Tracing 13 shows his pulse in a fully resting state. At the end of this tracing I heard someone asking for me in the adjacent room. Immediately afterward, the manservant entered and announced Prof. Lombroso.[7] At point α, tracing 14, I signaled while our colleague moved closer.

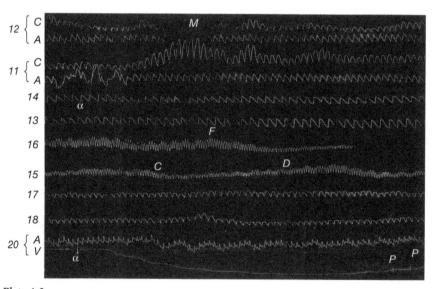

Plate 4.3

He looked at Mr. Bosio, the apparatus, and the tracing, upon which I pointed out to him the effect of his presence. Soon after he departed.

The alteration of the forearm pulse in line 14 is very conspicuous, although just what is most distinctive, namely, the volume change, one does not at all recognize in the tracing because the water of the hydrosphygmograph is in communication with the compensation surface. The contraction of the vessels is manifested (as was already stressed in another chapter) only by another position of the rise *S* and of the dicrotic elevation through which each pulse wave acquires a more peaked shape.

We have had occasion to see, together with Prof. Giacomini, other, no less interesting examples of such an influence of emotional excitement during our experiments with Catherina X. One day we were busy in the *Anatomicum* with the observations of the cerebral movements of this patient. Suddenly and without demonstrable external cause, we saw the height of the pulsations and the volume of the brain increase. The matter struck me as strange and I asked the woman how she felt. Catherina responded that she felt quite well. Since the high pulsations and the swelling of the brain did not subside, I interrupted the experiment to make sure all was in order with the apparatus, and then I asked the woman to tell me precisely and in detail what she might have thought about in the course of the last few minutes. She replied that she had at first been distracted, then had looked into the cabinet standing opposite her, where she saw a cranium; she became somewhat frightened by this skull, and in the course of this she also thought of her impending surgical operation.

On the alterations of the cerebral circulation based on contraction or relaxation of the cerebral vessels with increased mental activity, see Chapter 13.

NOTES

1. This is what people in Italy call a soup with any variety of vegetable ingredients.
2. A. Mosso: *Sopra un nuovo metodo per scrivere I movimenti dei vasi sanguigni dell' uomo*. R. Accad. delle scienze di Torino, 1875. Capitolo: *Sui movimenti dei vasi sanguigni che accompagnano le emozioni e l'attività del cerebrale*.
3. A. Mosso: *Die Diagnostik des Pulses*. Leipzig, 1879.
4. In the tracings obtained from Bertino, this phenomenon is less obvious, because the skin of his forearm was very hard and tanned by the sun, and his hands were callous from laboring in the fields.
5. Thanhoffer: *Der Einfluss der Gehirnthätigkeit auf den Puls*. Pflüger's Archiv, 1879, p. 225.
6. Franck: *Recherches critiques et expérimentales sur les mouvements alternatifs d'expansion et de resserrement du cerveau*. Journal de l'anatomie et de la physiologie de Ch. Robin, 1877, p. 301.
7. Trans.: Cesare Lombroso (1836–1909), known for his work on the biological determinism of criminality, was professor of medical law and psychiatry in Turin.

Sleep and Its Relationships to Cerebral Blood Flow

§. 5.1

Observations on Catherina X

Of all the investigations I have conducted on the circulation of the blood, these were the ones that I undertook with the keenest anticipation. Since, for years, I have had a particular predilection for studying the physiology of sleep, one will easily understand my special interest for this series of my hemodynamic observations and experiments.

Having already made the observation a few years ago that during the transition from the waking state to that of sleep, a slackening and widening of the forearm vessels take place, and that awakening is always accompanied by a contraction of the forearm vessels, and also, having postulated a mechanical theory according to which blood, upon awakening, is displaced from the extremities and is propelled toward the central organs of the nervous system in order to incite activity of these central organs, I finally had the opportunity to subject this theory to a direct experimental test.

I want to describe presently, without entering into any introductory reflections, the observations I performed on my three subjects with defects of cranial wall substance.

I obtained, together with Prof. Giacomini, the first of my recordings on Catherina X. in February of 1876. Of this patient I only have a few observations relative to normal sleep, for she had difficulty falling asleep in our presence, and when she did so, her sleep was so light that the slightest stimuli were enough to rouse her from it. The extraordinary width of the skull defect with which she was afflicted, and the difficulties that we encountered in these first experiments, prevented us from affording to our recording apparatus all the sensitivity that we could have achieved nowadays. It may therefore not surprise the reader to find that these tracings are not as characteristic as those obtained later on with little Thron, and especially those obtained finally with Bertino.

The patient was lying on her bed, her head propped up on a pillow, and the Marey cardiograph was attached to the skull defect in such a manner that its dome only just touched the scar that filled up the defect. Having made certain that the patient was sleeping, I woke her at the point shown in Fig. 5.1 tracing A. She opened her eyes and spoke, but soon after she seemed to have fallen asleep again.

About 15 minutes later, while she remained at complete rest and appeared to sleep, I touched her with my hand (tracing B, mark ⇓). She opened her eyes but did not move.

In these tracings as well as in several other experiments, which I omit for the sake of brevity, a slight increase in brain volume was noticeable at the moment of awakening.

However, since the patient's sleep was always very light and she did not easily fall asleep on her own, and since the experiments could only be conducted in the afternoon (when the patient was least inclined to go to sleep), we decided to resort to the use of chloral hydrate.

On March 1, 1876, at 2:57 in the afternoon, 1.50 of chloral hydrate, in water solution and with added syrup, was administered to the patient by mouth. Half an hour went by before she fell asleep. At 4 o'clock I woke her (tracing C, mark ⇓). She opened her eyes without speaking but did not go back to sleep. During this experiment we made the interesting observation that while the patient snored loudly, her pulse became more elevated, and that it became smaller again when she stopped snoring.

On the afternoon of March 10, 1876, at 2:40, we gave 2.0 of chloral hydrate to the patient and then halted the tracing of the cerebral pulse until 3:03. The patient had fallen into a deep sleep and was snoring. The pulse was very ample and the brain volume, as is visible in Plate 4.3, tracings 15 and 16, showed substantial swings. Breathing finally became so noisy that the patient woke up on her own because of it; or, rather, she conveyed that her sleep became lighter each time when, having been disturbed by excessively loud snoring, she returned to a more normal mode of respiration.

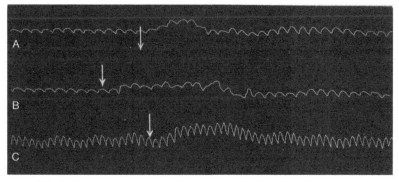

Figure 5.1 Modification of the cerebral pulse in Catherina X. at the moment she awakens. The moment is marked with an arrow. The rotational speed of the cylinder is less than in previous tracings. In tracing C, it is even lesser than in A and B.

The cerebral pulse in Plate 4.3, tracing 15, shows that during sleep, aside from individual pulsations, the oscillations related to respiratory movements as well as the undulations based on changes in the condition of the vessels and extending to longer periods also revealed themselves distinctly. The shorter length of the individual pulse waves, which is conspicuous in this tracing, was not, indeed, due to a greater pulse rate but only to the fact that the recording cylinder was rotating more slowly, whereby incidentally the fluctuations of brain volume also became much more visible.

As soon as the pulsations gained in amplitude, we noted that the patient began to snore. At the same time, the respiratory oscillations, too, became more distinct in the pulse tracing (Plate 4.3, lines 15 and 16). At point C the snoring diminished and one could see the tracing descend slightly. At D the patient started snoring again. At the beginning of line 16, the snoring was uncommonly loud and, accordingly, the heightening of the pulse quite extraordinary. In F the patient snored so loudly that she seemed to wake up on her own to return to an easier way of breathing. The pulse tracing descended and the individual pulsations became smaller; they remained at this lesser height for more than a minute, after which a second period of snoring began and the same phenomena repeated themselves.

One learns from the specified recordings that, in general, during the transition from sleep to the waking state, an increase in cerebral volume took place. The only negative result in this entire experimental series occurred when I tried to wake the patient at the very moment she stopped snoring on her own to return to a more superficial and quiet mode of respiration. Under those circumstances, any detectable alteration of the circulatory conditions in the brain failed to materialize twice in a row. This fact can be explained when one considers that snoring is imposed upon certain conditions that make the continuation of deep sleep impossible. Indeed, when the patient stopped snoring, a contraction of the cerebral vessels ensued. The cerebral volume diminished and the patient's sleep became so light that she woke up. On the face of it, it is difficult to decide which of the two phenomena represents the cause and which the effect. Nonetheless, in the case at hand, we may deem it very probable that in the course of touching the patient, and while she opened her eyes, the increase in brain volume failed to appear for the reason that, because of the preceding contraction of the vessels (during which the pulse tracing approached the abscissa), sleep had already become far too shallow.

§. 5.2

Observations on Thron During Sleep

Within a year I resumed these experiments, with prospects for better success, on little Thron. Yet I was strangely disappointed in this expectation when, during the night I had chosen for the first experiment in a hall of the insane asylum, I found the poor boy so fast asleep that I did not succeed in rousing him. Of all the experiments I have ever performed with human subjects, these have cost me the greatest effort and have left the most profound impression. I carried this out in conjunction with Dr. Albertotti. Since our experimental subject was a feebleminded boy, every small obstacle grew into enormous difficulties, so that even the application of the recording instruments was not always possible.[1]

If my results turned out less fortunate than I had expected, this is to be attributed to the state of mind of the small patient, specifically to his great agitation during the waking state, which in the first stage of the experiment prevented us nearly always from obtaining the normal tracing required in order to compare this to potential alterations of the pulse during sleep. Moreover, the frequent epileptic attacks that afflicted him in the last periods of his life contributed in no small measure to frustrate all our effort and care. His sleep was irregular, which is why during our nocturnal experiments we frequently found him awake at a late hour. He often suffered from insomnia, and in that case any measures by which we sought to procure sleep for him remained fruitless. Rather than arousal, it was instead nocturnal agitation that often presaged an epileptic attack. Even the administration of 2 g of chloral hydrate under such conditions did nothing but increase his excitability and failed to have a hypnotic effect. We often saw him seized by the most terrible epileptic spasms, and during the nights following such attacks his sleep became so profound and peculiar that one immediately understood this to be not a normal phenomenon but rather a morbid soporific condition: for one might shake the patient, stand him upright, call his name loudly, splash water on his face—all was to no avail in waking him from sleep for any length of time; he opened his eyes for a moment and immediately again fell into his slumber.

On April 23, 1877, Thron suffered a violent epileptic attack. When I visited him the next morning at 9 o'clock, he had fallen asleep. While the gutta percha plate was being applied to his head, he awoke but did not try, as he had on other occasions, to rip the instrument away from his head; he remained still for several minutes, during which time we prepared the tracing shown in Fig. 5.2. One can detect in this tracing quite manifestly the great influence that the respiratory movements exerted on the cerebral blood flow, even when they were not very profound.

Tracings 17 and 18 of Plate 4.3 were recorded on this same boy during sleep. Looking at the length of tracing 17 from one side, one can see that even at deepest rest there was still an influence of the respiratory movements on brain volume. Toward the middle of tracing 18, one can notice a substantial increase of the brain

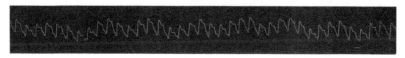

Figure 5.2 Thron. Cerebral pulse after an epileptic attack.

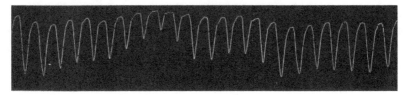

Figure 5.3 Thron. Alterations of the cerebral pulse during sleep.

volume, the cause of which remained unknown to me, even though I was observing the boy very carefully during this time (perhaps it was the effect of a dream image). The blunted peak of the individual pulsations, which one notices in these two tracings as well as in the three lines of the woodcut of Fig. 5.4, was merely due to the fact that the stylus was pushed too hard against the rotating cylinder and thus the characteristic shape of the peak of the pulse wave was smudged.

Here, too, as with Catherina X., marked fluctuations (undulations) of the cerebral pulse tracing became visible during sleep, with regular and not very deep breathing, when the pulsations might attain twice their previous height.

When sleep was induced by the action of chloral hydrate, we obtained very strong cerebral pulsations along with ample undulations, as one can see in Fig. 5.3.

Thron had had a violent epileptic attack at about 8 o'clock in the morning. Afterward, he was so dejected that he stayed in bed the whole day without having to be restrained, as was usually done to keep him quiet. At about 10 PM, we found him fast asleep. The skin overlying the skull defect was not very taut and pulsated strongly. We applied the gutta percha mold to the head after lightly warming its edges. The pulse depicted in the upper line of Fig. 5.4 can serve as a typical example for a long series of preliminary observations, which lasted without interruption for about 40 minutes. Afterward, we waited for another hour, and then, around 11 o'clock, we loudly called the young patient's name: "Giovanni." One can discern in the tracing (second line ⇓ G) that a perception—whether it was conscious or unconscious—had occurred here, which is why an increase in brain volume and an increase in amplitude of cerebral pulsations took place.

The following minute another voice repeated the same sound, and we called the patient's name in this manner several more times consecutively, in fact, always

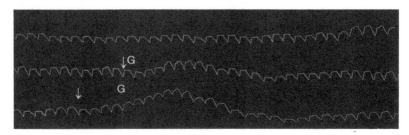

Figure 5.4 Thron. Cerebral pulse during sleep.

with interim minute-long pauses. The result was the same each time (Fig. 5.4, lower line, mark ⇓). This increase in brain volume was thus a constant phenomenon. Furthermore, it was not accompanied by any alteration of the cardiac rhythm and one must, in all probability, assume that it depended on the contraction of the vessels in the extremities and in other extracranial body parts, as we will more fully demonstrate later on.

§. 5.3

Observations on Caudana During Sleep

Although these experiments were imperfect in many respects, they were nevertheless sufficient to dampen the enthusiasm with which I had hypothesized and defended a mechanical theory of sleep in an earlier writing. Now, however, I had arrived at the conviction that the more forceful rush of blood to the brain, which takes place during the alert state and is based on the contraction of the peripheral vessels, constitutes only a concomitant phenomenon, and not the primary and essential condition of mental activity. By this time I was convinced that the weaker blood flow to the cerebral hemispheres was not the sole cause of sleep, but rather that, aside from alterations in circulatory conditions, there were other and even more substantial changes in the excitability and the nutritional state of the nervous centers, which must be the basis of sleep.

And yet, in spite of these disappointments (if such an expression is appropriate when more detailed investigations rectify a hasty conclusion, even if this, too, was drawn from objective observation), I detected beyond the question of the alterations of the cerebral blood circulation a field that was increasingly more interesting and worthy of investigation.

Indeed, the aforementioned observations were also enough to convince me that the physiology of sleep might cast a bright light onto certain psychological processes, and more particularly on the material conditions of consciousness.

This was the point of view from which I had carried out a series of observations on the variations of the forearm pulse during sleep, observations that may serve as an introduction to the much more complete and direct results gained from the study of Bertino's brain.

Tracing 1 on Plate 5.1 was obtained on Caudana's forearm while he was lying on a mattress and while I had been waiting for more than an hour for him to fall asleep. His pulse was highly irregular and in fact tricuspid, as is evident in the first line at the bottom. I omit, for the sake of brevity, the preceding 11 lines of my original plate (corresponding to as many minutes of observation), for they are all identical and do not show any modification of the pulse. During these experiments, my entire method consisted of an uninterrupted recording of the pulse that often lasted for 2 to 3 consecutive hours; it would therefore be both cumbersome and altogether useless to list the obtained recordings at this juncture, and this is why I also skip those of the next 10 minutes in order to arrive at line 2 of

Plate 5.1, where it became clear to me that in all likelihood Caudana had fallen asleep. Indeed, he did not move at all and his breathing had acquired the characteristics typical of sleep, when expiration is more rapid and somewhat noisy. The shape of the pulse changed, too, in that the arrangement of the three tips of the peak of the pulse wave had become less symmetric and less regular.

At point A, Caudana moved his right hand and scratched his chest. The irregularities appearing in the tracing at this moment were due to the fact that Caudana had tried to move his left hand, which was enclosed in the hydrosphygmograph. The pulse changed significantly. Instead of adopting the form I call tricuspid (with the highest tip in the middle), the three elevations of the wave peak decreased successively in amplitude and fell into the catacrotic wave leg.

I skip once more the tracing recorded by the next rotation of the kymograph barrel (which corresponds to 1 minute). In the meantime, the pulse returned to its original shape. Caudana did not stir any more. Line 3 represents this new period of quiet sleep. At the end of this line, while I was in the process of moving the stylus of the recording barrel upward to start the next line, I heard the slamming of the entrance door on the first floor near the portico. Caudana did not move and did not indicate in any way that he heard the sound; yet, the pulsations at his forearm underwent a marked change, very similar to the preceding one. In tracing 4 of Plate 5.1, the first eight pulsations are missing because the cylinder I used in these experiments had a greater circumference than the format of the figures cited here. At G, Caudana moved one of his feet, rubbing it against the other leg. At D in line 6, he started to speak and told me that he was awake. Immediately thereafter, the forearm pulse became smaller and more frequent (line 7). In the next line (line 8) the forearm pulse returned to its normal shape, typical of sleep. At E, Caudana asked me to cover his face with a towel so that he might fall asleep more easily.

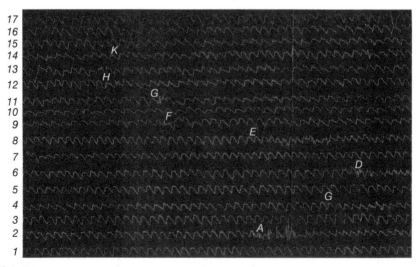

Plate 5.1

Ten minutes went by, and then slight muscle twitches happened at brief intervals, such as they occur in all people during sleep and which are frequently apt to interrupt sleep. I continued recording the pulse. Lines 9 to 12 represent a fragment of the page being inscribed half an hour after Caudana had spoken. His sleep was deep, and the alteration of the pulse was so prominent that I need not point this out explicitly. In 9 *F*, 11 *G*, and 12 *H*, another few muscle twitches occurred. After these movements, the contour of the pulse changed, as one sees in *G* and *H*, and took a shape that suggested a contraction of the blood vessels. This phenomenon was much more apparent after the mark *K* in line 15, where I wound the Breguet clockwork of the instrument. This manipulation lasted about 20 seconds and was accompanied by a noise. During this time, the profile of the pulsations indicated strong contraction of the vessels. Caudana did not signal in any way that he might be awake. At the beginning of line 14 and at the position marked *K* of line 16, a transformation of the forearm pulse ensued yet again, the cause for which remains unknown to me.

As opposed to the behavior of the pulse during the waking state, the continuous variability of the condition of the vessels during Caudana's sleep was most especially striking. Even though I can in no way pose such a pulse configuration as the rule (for elsewhere, in cases of the most profound sleep, I also observed a very regular forearm pulse), I have deemed it appropriate to mention these very tracings for reasons to be clarified later on (see Chapter 6).

§. 5.4

Observations on Bertino During Sleep

Now I shall follow up in chronological sequence with some of the observations that I carried out on Bertino with regard to the manifestations of sleep.

The first of these observations took place on the evening of September 24, 1877. At 8:15 PM, Bertino lay down on a sofa with his head propped up and his body wrapped in a blanket. I had previously applied the gutta percha plate to his head and repeatedly explained the purpose of the experiments, with the request for him to remain completely still and to fall asleep as quickly as possible. His replies demonstrated that he was not at all convinced of the usefulness of such observations, and we feared that because of his suspicious mood he might not fall asleep easily.

After about an hour I inscribed line 1 on Plate 5.2. I was convinced that Bertino was not asleep: the pulsations were very strong and tricuspid. The man remained very still, but another hour went by without him falling asleep. The pulse, as can be seen on Plate 5.2, line 2, diminished somewhat. A few minutes later Bertino took a deep breath and moved his hands as though he wanted to stretch, as one does when yawning; in so doing he opened his eyes and asked me whether he had already slept for a long time. As the sincerity of this question appeared to be dubious to me (for in listening attentively to his

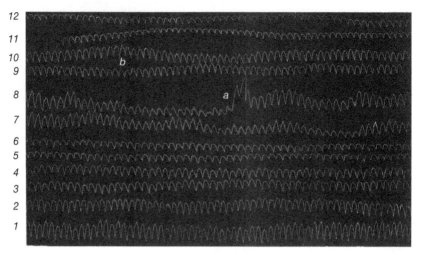

Plate 5.2

respirations I had not at all been convinced that he was asleep), I responded evasively, saying that it had not yet been enough, and asked him to go back to sleep; I also added the remark that I would not let him go at all unless he had been truly fast asleep.

Yet another hour went by, during which now and then I recorded the pulse. Bertino remained completely motionless. The brain volume showed prominent undulations as is seen in lines 3 and 4, which I recorded at 11:03 PM The pulsations were lower and smaller than before. I let pass another quarter of an hour and then wrote, at 11:45, lines 5 and 6 of Plate 5.2, where one can see that the cerebral vessels showed some unrest although respiration was even and superficial. After completion of these two lines, I called Bertino's name. He moved his head immediately and started to speak, telling me that he was asleep. These movements distorted the tracing to such a degree that I could not reproduce this point of the observation. Lines 7 and 8 represent the tracings of the cerebral pulse, which were achieved 4 minutes after Bertino's full arousal.

In *a*, tracing 8, Bertino told me that he feared he might not be able to fall asleep. Here, as in earlier observations, we have another beautiful example of the marked volume increase of the brain and of the increase in amplitude of its pulsations under the influence of psychic movement.

Around midnight, when Bertino made clear to us that he would most likely not be able to fall fast asleep the entire night because, he said, he was far too nervous, we broke off the session.

While we deem this observation unreliable with respect to sleep, which in any case must have been very light, we can see nevertheless how the pulse underwent strong variations during the transition from alertness to deep rest, and how the blood flow in the brain again became irregular and the pulsations of this organ stronger as soon as mental activity was fully restored.

These successive transformations of the pulse during transition from the waking state to complete rest and sleep could also be discerned in all later series of our nocturnal observations.

Here, for example, was Bertino's pulse at 8 PM the next evening, while he maintained the same position as on the previous evening.

These two tracings (9 and 10, Plate 5.2) were obtained while Bertino had been lying on the sofa very still and with his eyes closed for a quarter of an hour. The general tracing shows strong undulations and the shape of the pulse is tricuspid. The irregularity noted on pulsation *b* of line 10 derives from the egress of an air bubble from the Müllerian valve (thus from an increase in pressure). Another half an hour later, at 8:45, the pulse shape had already changed: the pulse was less ample and more regular.

I do not present an example of the sphygmograms obtained during this time, which revealed a very regular sequence of pulsations, and provide only two lines that were obtained successively and reveal strong undulations (11 and 12, Plate 5.2).

At the start of line 11, Plate 5.2, Dr. De Paoli entered the room. As soon as I heard the door open, I set the cylinder into motion and recorded the strong undulation, which can be observed at the beginning of this line: the entire curve rises very markedly (therefore, significant volume increase of the brain), while its individual pulse waves lose height noticeably. The reason for the undulations visible in line 12 is unknown to me. Upon awakening, Bertino told me he had not noticed at all that someone had entered the room.

———————————

I omit the pulse tracings obtained during the following 14 minutes; at 9:30, tracing 13, Plate 5.3 was recorded. If we compare this pulse image to the previous ones, we see that the cerebral pulsations decreased in height to the extent

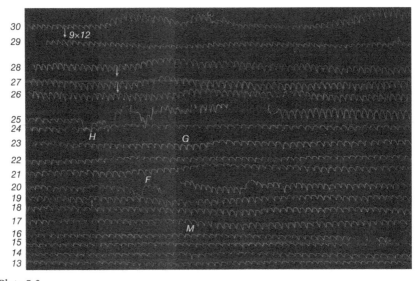

Plate 5.3

that sleep became deeper. The wide oscillations that we observed during waking faded; the pulse was more even. The consecutively recorded tracings in lines 13, 14, 15, and 16 show by their almost horizontal configuration and their highly regular, uniform shape that the cerebral vessels were in a state of deep repose. Now and then, however, Bertino took a deep breath, upon which followed a slight diminution of the cerebral volume (see place *M* in line 17). What is more, the pulse rate dropped, whereby the pulsations took on a distinct tricuspid contour. For approximately a quarter of an hour, brain volume and brain pulse remained unchanged, except for the previously mentioned slight fluctuations after deep inspirations. The cerebral pulse tracing runs horizontally without definite undulations. After line 17, I had stopped the cylinder.

In the meantime, I heard the hospital clock strike 10. I do not know to what extent this sound was responsible for the transformation we detected in the cerebral pulse tracings of the lines following thereupon.

In tracing 19 of Plate 5.3, there is a question mark at the beginning of the line. This is a notation I made because I could not account for the successive amplitude increase of the pulsations, which indicated an imminent awakening. As a matter of fact, while line 20 was being registered, Bertino scratched himself and moved his head and legs. He did not, however, open his eyes. A minute later, tracing 21, at point *F*, I inquired softly whether he was sleeping. He did not stir and did not respond with any sound, but there was an increase in volume detectable in the brain. I let another 2 minutes go by and then, to make certain that he was awake, I touched his face lightly with the stylus (at point *G*, tracing 23). Bertino did not move but the volume of his brain increased immediately and the contour of its pulsations changed. In the next line, he turned his head on the pillow. At first the pulsations augmented, and then they diminished again. The respiration behaved as is usual during sleep.

At 10:30 (point *H*, at the beginning of tracing 24), I said in a loud voice: "*Bertino, è finito*" (we have finished). He did not stir. In the course of the next line (line 25), while I would the Breguet clockwork of the recording apparatus, Bertino woke up and repeatedly moved his head and arms, which distorted the tracing. Since we had reached the last line, the stylus lost contact with the cylinder. I was required to vent the release flap (clarinet).

A few seconds later I was able to resume recording and discovered that the cerebral pulsations had reverted to their original configuration, the same as in the waking state at the start of the experiment. I immediately inspected the man's eyes and recognized from the reddening of the conjunctiva that he had really been asleep.

———————————

On the evening of September 27, we undertook with Bertino a new series of observations concerning the behavior of the cerebral circulation during sleep. At 8 o'clock, he lay down on the sofa, and an hour later he had fallen into a light slumber. This time his pulse was clearly catacrotic, in contrast to the previous evenings. To be concise, I limit myself to describing only a few lines of the tracings obtained in that session.

Here, too, exterior stimuli, even when slight, caused major alterations of the cerebral blood circulation and of the pulse configuration. At 9:02, I noticed that Bertino's breathing was very shallow. After recording the first eight pulsations of the engraving of Fig. 5.5 I tried to ascertain whether he was really sleeping: I stood up and called his name (at the mark ⇓). Bertino did not stir and did not reply. Upon inspection of this tracing, we saw that before the mark ⇓, four pulsations were already somewhat higher than the preceding ones. This is probably due to the slight noise I generated when I stood up and approached Bertino's ear. While I called his name, there were three more normally shaped pulsations, and then the brain volume increased and the pulsations became anacrotic and retained this configuration for more than a minute. One only needs to compare the beginning and the end of Fig. 5.5 to appreciate that extensive transformations of the pulse took place during sleep, without their inducing causes leaving the slightest trace in the sleeper's memory. The previously catacrotic pulsations had become anacrotic. The blood flow to the brain was augmented, and for about 30 seconds the volume of the organ stayed greater than the preceding, as one can easily substantiate in Fig. 5.5 when measuring the vertical distance from the abscissa of the base of the individual pulse waves.

I continued recording the cerebral pulsations for another quarter of an hour. During this period of time the volume of the brain showed intermittent fluctuations, which were independent of the respiratory movements. On my original plate these are labeled with a question mark since I could not relate them to any demonstrable exterior source. They might have stemmed from inner causes, dreams, or other causative factors unbeknownst to me. Line 26 of Plate 5.3 (the further continuation of the same evening session to which the engraving of Fig. 5.5 refers) offers an example of such spontaneous undulations of the cerebral tracing.

Immediately following this line and without stopping the kymograph, I inscribed line 27. At the location of mark ⇓, I spoke softly into Bertino's ear: "*Dormite, Bertino?*" ("Are you sleeping?"). A slight volume increase of the brain ensued; however, the man did not stir and did not show in any way that he had awakened. Breathing was deep, and expiration was accompanied by a slight noise, as is usually the case during sleep. The pulse became tricuspid. In the following minute, tracing 28, mark ⇓, I repeated the same question without Bertino's awakening. The changes in the cerebral circulation were the same.

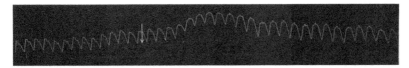

Figure 5.5 Modification of the cerebral pulse in Bertino, after he was called at point ⇓, without having awakened.

Due to space constraints, I do not reproduce a series of subsequent tracings and restrict myself to a brief description of the phenomena observed.

Another minute passed, following which Bertino took in two rather deep breaths. The cerebral volume decreased so much that I was required to vent the relief valve (clarinet) to bring the pressure within the recording barrel back to 0. A distortion of the pulse tracing followed. During the next 20 seconds, the breaths were again normal and shallow, whereupon followed another deep inspiration. The pulse waves became more catacrotic and the pulse tracing narrower.

Soon after, I noticed a slight but rapid increase of the brain volume: Bertino woke up and opened his eyes. Twenty seconds went by, during which time the pulse tracing, because of the displacements of the head, adopted an irregular shape; I then asked the man whether he was unable to sleep. He replied that he had a dream and told me a muddled story in which the most interesting detail was that his village priest had called his name; more precisely, it was my call that had interfered in an already emerged and developing web of dreams and was interpreted as the voice of the village priest.

Shortly afterward, in tracing 29 of Plate 5.3, the height of the pulse diminished for no reason known to me. In order to be sure that the man was fully awake, I asked him (tracing 30, at the position of the ⇓) how many eggs were in nine dozen. The subsequent, stronger, rush of blood to the brain was extremely characteristic and corresponded to the examples communicated in the preceding chapter. The second increase in volume corresponded to the point in time when Bertino responded "one hundred eight." Toward the end of the line, a marked increase of pulse amplitude and cerebral volume became apparent again, which I must construe as the after-effect of the cerebral effort during the suddenly undertaken mental operation. A second multiplication, which the man performed later, produced an even stronger primary flow of blood to the brain but did not result in any added delayed change.

At 10 o'clock, while I was recording the last line of tracing, Bertino spontaneously took a deep inspiration, which was followed by a very significant decrease of the brain volume.

§. 5.5

Chloral Hydrate–Induced Sleep

At 8:20 PM on the evening of September 29, I undertook with Bertino another series of experiments on sleep, which was to be the last, since a few days later the man suddenly left the hospital to return to his family.

After the gutta percha plate had been fastened to his forehead, Bertino lay down on the sofa, and I started, as I did during the previous sessions, to record the cerebral pulse. Since the reproduction of all the tracings recorded in the course of this approximately 3-hour session, which take up four large pages in my original collection, would occupy an inordinate amount of space, I will leave out those of the first hour and only mention in writing the most salient points to be noted on these omitted plates.

The cerebral pulse was at first rather small and catacrotic. After a 10-minute observation, I turned to Dr. De Paoli and told him that we had better administer the tranquillizer (calmante) to Bertino right away so that he might sleep better. Although Bertino had been informed beforehand that he was to take chloral hydrate, he still seemed to be somewhat upset by these words: indeed, soon afterward his brain volume increased and the pulsations became higher.

While the recording of the subsequent line proceeded, Bertino drained the aqueous solution of chloral hydrate (with added syrup). Immediately afterward, the pulse became smaller. This was a manifestation of the cerebral pulse we want to make note of here, and which also proves to be constant for the forearm pulse, no matter what medication is taken. The concomitant vascular contraction is all the more pronounced the more unpleasant the taste of the medication swallowed. In the case at hand, it did not escape our notice that the patient was very reluctant to take the medicine even though he did not say anything about it.

Thirty minutes later he had not yet fallen asleep. At 9 o'clock, given the characteristics of his respiratory movements, it seemed to me that sleep had already set in. The cerebral volume displayed undulations. I succeeded in verifying that some of these followed upon several deeper respiratory movements; for others, the cause remained unknown to me, and I therefore designate the latter as **spontaneous fluctuations**. On several occasions, in order to examine changes in the receptivity for exterior stimuli during sleep, I produced a slight noise by tapping on the table with the interphalangeal joint of my index finger: on each of these occasions, a volume increase of the brain ensued and the shape of the pulse underwent a slight alteration similar to that we saw in the earlier examples. Meanwhile, Bertino did not stir, even when I softly called his name.

Line 1 of Fig. 5.6 shows the configuration of the cerebral pulse during sleep. In line 2, at point *B*, I called the man's name out loudly. He woke up and moved his hands and his head. In this case, according to the tracing, volume increase of the brain during the transition from sleep to waking was missing; in fact, there was a diminution of the intracranial blood content instead. A detriment, which I could not redress in any way during these experiments, consists in the involuntary movements of the head, the trunk, and the extremities at the moment of awakening. Naturally, it is difficult to evaluate properly a decrease of the cerebral tracing

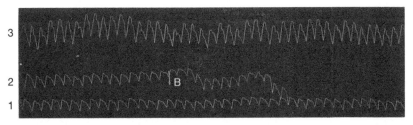

Figure 5.6 **Line 1**. Cerebral pulse during chloral hydrate sleep. **Line 2**. Ibid. **Line 3**. Cerebral pulse immediately after awakening.

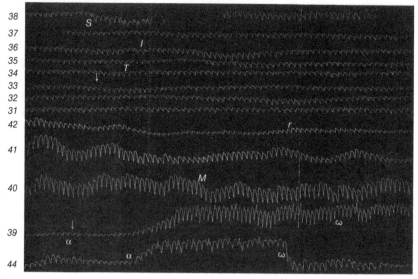

Plate 5.4

under such circumstances, for it is brought about under the influence of several heterologous effects. Be that as it may, we must remember the fact that in the present case, a diminution of the blood content of the cerebral hemispheres took place on awakening. Later, at the instance of an analogous example, I will return to this subject; for now, I only note that after about 15 seconds the brain became more voluminous than before, and that during the waking state its pulsations were twice as high as during sleep (see the upper line 3 of the tracing in Fig. 5.6).

At the end of this partial observation I stood up, viewed the tracings obtained, and started to blacken two new cylinders whereby I attempted to make as little noise as possible. In the meantime, Bertino went back to sleep. For about a half an hour, I recorded the cerebral pulse without interruption. The tracings appeared very regular (line 31, Plate 5.4); nevertheless, intermittent undulations occurred, which seemed to stem from a decrease in the frequency of the cardiac beats (see second half of line 32 and first half of line 33 on Plate 5.4). The ideal baseline of the curve fell with regard to the abscissa, and the entire tracing underwent a general drop. This decrease in volume may stem from a deeper inspiratory movement, which I must have missed. At least this is really the case in line 36 of Plate 5.4, which was inscribed approximately a quarter of an hour later: I noticed that Bertino in his sleep took a deep breath; I immediately carved the mark I above the pulse tracing, and soon thereafter a volume decrease of the brain and a lessening of the rate of the heartbeats ensued. The physiognomy of this fluctuation is analogous to those of the swings in lines 32 and 33.

Yet, apart from this great similarity, I repeat that I lack sufficient positive data to attribute the variations of these latter lines to the same causal moment as that of line 36. This caution in interpretation seems to me all the more necessary as I encountered such variations of pulse rate and brain volume on several occasions, at times when I had determined with certainty the perfect regularity of the respiratory movements. Oftentimes I have also observed very similar alterations of the cerebral tracings under the influence of exterior causes. In line 34, I coughed very softly at point ⇓. The volume increase of the brain was barely noticeable. I did not stop the cylinder, and in the next minute, in T of line 35, I touched Bertino's ear very lightly with the stylus. A slight increase in brain volume and in cardiac frequency followed, whereupon a decrease of the cerebral volume and pulse rate set in. On the basis of this observation as well as of other, similar ones, which I will not mention for the sake of brevity, I deem it probable that some of the undulations of the brain were controlled by the force and frequency of the heartbeats, and this independently of the respiratory movements.

Bertino did not wake up. A normal pulse tracing followed, line 37, in which no undulation was noted. In the next line (line 38), which is the last, I scratched the mark S into the blackened paper of the cylinder. As soon as the stylus reached this mark, I called out Bertino's name and he awoke immediately. Since I had not called out loudly and since he opened his eyes right away, one may well assume that his sleep was no longer deep. The tracing curve fell; thus, in waking, the brain experienced once more a decrease in volume instead of an increase. True, here, too, a movement of the head and trunk had followed immediately after waking up. So that the tracing should not descend to the preceding line, I lifted the relief valve (clarinet) and in this way I brought the pressure in the recording barrel back to zero. However, as soon as this had taken place, I noticed that the brain quickly swelled again and I had to vent the valve once more. This manipulation, which I was forced to repeat in all my experiments whenever Bertino woke up, made it a priori impossible for me to determine the exact point in time when, after the relaxation of the primary vascular contraction, the brain returned to its original volume and by how much it surpassed this.

At the same time, these observations elucidate most definitely that in the first moment of awakening, the brain can under certain circumstances undergo a volume decrease and thus in fact comprise less blood than during sleep,; this is perfectly sufficient to demonstrate the fallacy of the assumption that sleep is based on ischemia of the brain.

NOTES

1. I take with pleasure this opportunity to express my warmest gratitude to the direction of the local insane asylum, which sought to facilitate my experiments in every way, and most especially to the Messrs. Drs. Perotti, Albertotti, and Valetti, who took a lively interest in them.

6

Reflections on the Nature of Sleep and Its Concomitant Phenomena

§. 6.1

In the preceding chapter, we saw that during the transition from waking to deep rest, and from this to sleep, the blood circulation in the brain undergoes successive alterations. We will now subject the factual findings to a general review and attempt, if possible, to relate them to each other. During sleep, a dilatation of the vessels takes place in the extremities, which in man we have been able to monitor through the plethysmographic measurement of the variations in volume of the forearm. The hydrosphygmographic observations on the contour of the pulse then undertaken have confirmed the corresponding slackening of the vascular walls. Every external excitation effects a contraction of the forearm vessels together with a consecutive increase of blood pressure, which results in augmented blood flow to the brain. Even though the cerebral vessels may contract as happens during sudden awakening, the general increase in blood pressure nonetheless produces an acceleration of the bloodstream in the cerebral hemispheres.

The frequency of the heartbeats diminishes somewhat during the transition from waking to sleep. Yet, this is a phenomenon that, when one inspects the pulse tracings, is the least conspicuous. If one compares the number of pulsations per 30 seconds in the different pulse tracings, there is, during sleep, on average, a decrease in frequency of three or four beats. However, if one correlates frequency with a smaller temporal unit, the result can be uncertain, because the rhythm of cardiac movements, as we have seen repeatedly in our observations, undergoes very substantial fluctuations during sleep.

The same changes that in the waking state are produced by mental activity in our body also repeat themselves during sleep through external influences upon our sensory organs, even when such influences are unable to awaken us from sleep.

We have seen that the sound of a voice, a noise, a touch, the effect of light, or, in short, any external sensory stimulus is capable of changing the rhythm of breathing to bring about contraction of the forearm vessels, increase in blood pressure, and intensification of blood flow to the brain, and to heighten the frequency of the heartbeats. If at the moment we notice these functional variations we allow a second influence to take effect, which will interrupt sleep, and if then we immediately ask the subject of observation regarding the content of his consciousness, the answer we get in the majority of cases is that sleep had been very profound and that there remained no memory of the outer influences received in the course of sleep. Nonetheless, on some occasions the external influences reach conscious perception and elicit dream imagery or are integrated into already developing dreams. Yet in both cases, the exact recognition of the perceived outer stimuli is missing, and as the latter are elaborated into dream images, they are so distorted that even on instant waking the subject can no longer grasp their true origin and their significance.

Among the modifications of the blood flow caused by unconscious events, we have until now considered only two kinds: namely, those stemming from external stimuli and others following upon more forceful respiratory movements. However, in the course of the first plethysmographic investigations I conducted on the activity of the blood circulation during sleep starting in 1874, I already noticed that there are movements in the vessels of the forearm that are controlled neither by unusually forceful breaths nor by any other demonstrable external influences, and which I have designated as **spontaneous**.

By means of hydrosphygmographic observation I have since then been able to witness how, together with volume changes of the forearm (already detected earlier with the help of the plethysmograph), the configuration of the pulse, too, varies during sleep, but even during this series of observations, and in spite of all precautions, the spontaneous vascular movements, the origin of which I was unable to explain, surfaced time and again. Excluding the influence of outer stimuli and of respiratory movements, their source could only be found in internal processes of the organism.

I initially assumed that these unregulated circulatory swings might be dependent on dreams that emerge during sleep. I tried to wake the persons subjected to observation, and it appeared now and then that they had indeed been dreaming. However, in the majority of cases, I did not receive an answer indicative of a dream or of another perception, even when sleep was interrupted at the very instant that the vascular contraction had set in. Thus, in such cases the vascular contraction was no doubt independent of conscious psychic events. Yet its frequently analogous behavior, as in cases when it was demonstrably correlated to such events, makes it for me very probable that even here it was not only the cerebral events themselves but also psychic-cerebral activities (i.e., excitations of the psychic centers that were unconscious) that acted as the cause.

That there are unconscious psychic processes during sleep as well as in the waking state has long been recognized in psychophysiology. In Lotze (in Wagner's *Handw. der Physiol.* III, I), we find a cursory mention of such processes. Carpenter is very explicit on the subject. Among the newest authors we find the following passage in Maudsley's *Physiology of the Mind*[1]:

If an idea fades from the conscious mind, it is not necessary for it to disappear from it completely; it can remain latent beneath the horizon (under the threshold) of consciousness, while the streams of molecular motion lessen by and by until this motion completely fades/subsides. Moreover, in remaining active beneath the horizon of consciousness, the same idea can exert an influence on this movement and on other ideas. For once we discover that the same effect we know to have been the conscious product of an idea, is also produced unconsciously, we appropriately conclude that a similar causative factor must have been active, all the more so since it sometimes happens that when our awareness is suddenly distracted from its operations, or from something which earlier on occupied its sphere, we capture the unconscious idea in its very act. The existence of a certain energy and intensity within the sphere of imagination will undoubtedly be manifest as the condition of consciousness.

This doctrine of the unconscious activity of the conceptual centers, which at first glance seems unacceptable as though it implied the assumption of a labor lost—a useless consumption of energy when conceptual activity takes place without consciousness—has the great advantage to explain many psychological facts, for which up until now a more satisfactory interpretation was lacking. I will not further pursue this subject and will only add that while my investigations on sleep can be interpreted in the sense of Maudsley's theory, on the other hand, they support the assumption that during sleep there is a period of such profound rest of the psychic centers that in it all conceptual activity, even the unconscious one, comes to a complete halt. To such a period would correspond those portions of the pulse tracings in which the pulse contours become regular and uniform.

§. 6.2

The study of the variations that the blood circulation in the brain and in the extremities undergoes during sleep cannot be separated from that of the corresponding variations of the respiratory system, for the individual parts of our body are so closely linked to one another that a change in the mechanisms of one immediately generates changes in the functions of the others. Thus, in our graphic images of sleep, we have often seen that an involuntary deep inspiration corresponded to a volume diminution of the brain and of the forearm, and that the vascular contraction altered the pulse contour of these organs (Fig. 6.1).

The variations of the rhythm and shape of the respiratory movements constitute a very interesting chapter in the physiology of sleep. I have already dealt with this subject in an earlier work[2] and return to this only to add some new observations necessary for the understanding of the questions occupying us here.

During sleep, the respiratory movements undergo unconscious modifications, analogous to those we have already become acquainted with in the blood

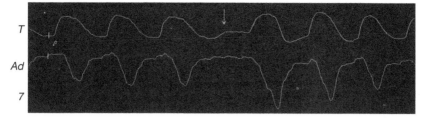

Figure 6.1 Respiratory movements during sleep. *T*. Tracing of thoracic respiration. *Ad*. Tracing of the abdominal respiration recorded simultaneously. The arrow corresponds to a noise, which did not wake the sleeper. NB. The thoracic tracing is inverted; that is, it falls during expansion of the thorax and rises with its falling. The abdominal tracing, on the other hand, represents the excursions of the abdominal wall in a direct illustration.

circulation of the brain and forearm. As examples I cite some pertinent tracings to follow.

The respiratory movements of the thorax were recorded with a Marey pneumograph; this is why tracing *T* represents an inverted image of these movements: it sinks with the inspiratory rise and rises with the expiratory falling of the thorax. In contrast, the abdominal tracing *Ad* was obtained by means of a barrel, the knob of which was set on the skin in the vicinity of the umbilicus: it rises with the lifting and sinks with the falling of the abdominal wall.

Caudana had sunk into a deep sleep. Corresponding to the mark ⇓ in Fig. 6.1, when I coughed involuntarily, the respiratory sequence changed suddenly even though Caudana had otherwise not stirred at all. During our inspection of the respiratory tracings, we noticed that a short pause ensued in the already begun expiratory movement and that the respiratory tracing was somewhat more markedly inclined toward the right than the preceding ones.

Thereafter, a deeper and more rapid inspiration followed; then there was, as it were, a slow start of expiratory movement, upon which there again followed an expiration stronger than the preceding ones. One look at the tracings was enough to persuade oneself that the respiratory movements of the thorax and of the abdominal wall had really become more powerful. I continued for another 20 seconds approximately with the recording of the respiratory movements, and then called Caudana's name (Fig. 6.2, mark ⇓). An immediate pause ensued, and shortly afterward a profound transformation of the respiratory motion set in. Caudana opened his eyes a few seconds after the inscription of the last respirations in Fig. 6.2. I asked him whether he heard me cough; he replied that he knew nothing of it, that he was sleeping and did not have any dreams. Let us review this recording once more from the start and inspect it carefully in order to survey the entire series of transformations the respiratory movements underwent during sleep, specifically since the auditory stimulus, which Caudana, when I woke him less than a minute later, stated not having heard at all. First, we made sure that the two writing styli, as indicated by the orientation bar *P*, were precisely aligned vertically.

The first thing we noticed here was the complete lack of parallelism between the respiratory movements of the thorax and those of the abdominal wall. Indeed, at the moment when the thorax performed the expiratory motion, the soft abdominal wall rose (see, e.g., Fig. 6.2, slightly to the right of *p*). And when the inspiratory motion of the thorax began, conversely, a simultaneous lowering of the soft abdominal layers followed. I already explained this lack of parallelism between the respiratory movements of the thorax and of the abdominal wall, which at first glance may seem paradoxical, in my treatise cited previously.[3] The reason for this phenomenon lies in the fact that the diaphragm, having been throughout the day and generally in the waking state the most intensely active of the respiratory muscles, reduces its activity during sleep. In the waking state, the abdomen rises with the expansion of the thorax because the diaphragm falls simultaneously with the contraction of the intercostal muscles. But when, for some reason, the inspiratory movement of the thorax becomes dominant, or the contraction of the diaphragm becomes weaker, then the abdomen must necessarily sink together with the expansion of the thorax, because this creates substantial space in the hypochondria, which the abdominal viscera are compelled to fill up (Hutchinson, following a citation of Ludwig). Yet, since during sleep the inspiratory fall of the soft abdominal layers is not based on strengthened expansion of the thorax but just on the weakened activity of the diaphragm, we infer from this that the thoracic excursions are in no way more extensive during sleep, but that the global excursions of the abdominal layers seem distinctly less important than in the waking state, and moreover, as my further investigations have shown,[4] that the amount of air taken in with each inspiration is significantly diminished.[5] In the course of inspiration, however, the activity of the diaphragm reawakens. We cannot assume that the contraction is able to take it far beyond its resting state, for in the subsequent expiration, the abdomen remains immobile, and at times, as can be seen in the second tracing, rather than falling, it is instead propelled slightly upward by the positive pressure created with thoracic expiration.

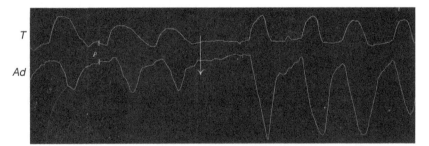

Figure 6.2 Variations of the thoracic and abdominal respirations (*T* and *Ad*) at the moment ⇓ when the sleeper was awakened. NB. The thoracic tracing is inverted; that is, it sinks during expansion of the thorax and rises with its falling. The abdominal tracing, on the other hand, represents the excursions in direct illustration.

These facts demonstrate that, during sleep, thoracic respiration prevails and that the diaphragm forfeits its energy to such an extent that it only follows the respiratory movements of the thorax, almost like a sluggish membrane.

As soon as a sound occurred, the rhythm and force of the diaphragmatic respiration changed, immediately and without participation of will or consciousness, to become more active. The modifications of diaphragmatic activity are much more evident in the second tracing, where I called Caudana's name. The moment I uttered the name Agostino, the breathing movement immediately stopped and then, as before, a deeper expiration ensued.

The diaphragm abandoned its inactivity and resumed its contractions in unison with the accessory respiratory muscles. Indeed, we see that the abdominal and thoracic tracings in both respiratory phases were more precisely concordant than earlier, and that expiration occurred simultaneously in the thorax and the abdomen. The slight deviation that still existed between the onset of the thoracic and abdominal inspiration disappeared in tracing 28, as soon as Caudana had time to wake up completely. A circumstance that is striking when one considers these tracings is the significant modification they undergo during transition from sleep to waking. The almost exclusively thoracic respiration of sleep was transformed during waking into a nearly pure diaphragmatic one.

This phenomenon, which I have termed **alternation of the respiratory movements, of the diaphragm, and of the thorax**, will soon be of service for our further observations on the nature of sleep: a priori we keep hold of the fact that external impressions are able to change respiration very substantially without thereby interrupting sleep, and that during sleep a series of unconscious impressions are registered, which can alter the functions of the organism very significantly without leaving a trace in the memory.

§. 6.3

These alterations occurring without our knowledge constitute one of the most wonderful systems that we may be able to observe amid the perfections of our organization. During the interruption of consciousness, our body is not helplessly exposed to the influences of the outside world or left in danger of falling prey to its enemies. Even during sleep, a part of the nervous center monitors the influences of the external world, and prepares in a timely manner the material conditions for the awakening of consciousness. If we review the unconscious processes we saw unfold under external influences during sleep, it becomes evident to us that they are all coordinated toward a final result: all concur in a final outcome that promotes blood circulation in the brain and thereby makes it possible, in case of danger, for the organ to wake up to full function.

I do not believe that I am far from the truth in declaring that the sum of the reflex movements that can be observed during sleep constitutes a veritable defense apparatus for the organism. Since here we find ourselves in a little-explored field of physiology, I may be permitted, with the guide of modern theories, to revisit the origin of this alternation of rest and activity of the nervous centers, of which sleep and waking consist.

Spencer correctly remarked in his *Principles of Physiology* [sic[6]]:[7]

> ... that if life were monotone and the cosmic conditions such that influences of any kind could be exerted equally at any time, restitution and consumption in all organs, including the nervous centers, would take place in approximately equal manner. Meanwhile, the alternation of day and night brings with it an alternation of greater and of lesser performance capacity, the effect of which in organisms adapting to that change is manifested by a sequence of exhaustion and recovery. This adaptation occurs through the fact that the more adaptable organisms survive the less adaptable ones. An animal constituted in such a way that within it, in the course of twenty-four hours, consumption and replacement were always in balance, would under otherwise equal circumstances be defeated by an enemy or rival who in the night hours, during which he retires, might only be capable of a lesser act of strength, yet under the favorable influence of daylight might be able to develop greater energy. So it was that the rhythmic alternation of nervous activity which we call sleep and waking, must necessarily have come about.

We know from our own experience that the effect of sleep is all the more refreshing the deeper it is, and that conversely, the mind's unrest prevents restorative sleep.

If we agree with Spencer's views on the origin of sleep, we must conclude that the ideal organism, one that makes the greatest possible use of its strengths, will be all the more perfect the more quickly it is able to recover during the night for renewed achievement, by yielding without any anxiety to deep sleep.

In our body we find these conditions to be realized in a wonderfully simple manner.

After the efforts of the day, man seeks a resting place and falls asleep. The muscles of the extremities, trunk, and neck slacken completely. The eyelids drop and cover the eye. The breathing sequence changes, and while respiration during waking is predominantly diaphragmatic, during sleep it becomes almost exclusively thoracic. Relaxation of the diaphragm can become so significant that this muscle appears to be completely inactive. The processes of combustion within the organism are so slowed down that instead of the 7 liters per minute inspired during waking, now only 1 liter per minute is absorbed. The force and frequency of the heartbeats are diminished; the vessels dilate, the blood pressure decreases, and the body temperature falls markedly.

Yet, during this state of profound sleep, there is an entire system of nerve fibers and ganglion cells that continues to function and monitors the influences of the external environment. A sound, a distant noise, a ray of light penetrating through the eyelids, a soft touch, or any other external influence is enough for respiration to become instantly active, for the vessels of the extracephalic organs to contract, for the heartbeats to become stronger and more frequent, for the blood pressure to rise, and for blood to flow more abundantly to the brain. With these material conditions for consciousness put into place, it is clear that the body, during its struggle for existence, will be able to escape the harmful influences of the environment all the more readily the more fully and perfectly it carries out this unconscious surveillance of external stimuli, thus allowing the psychic centers to move rapidly from deep repose to full action before danger is too near and harm becomes inevitable.

NOTES

1. Maudsley: *The Physiology of [the] Mind*. London, 1876, p. 305.
2. Mosso: *Sul polso negativo e sui rapporti della respirazione addominale e toracica nell'uomo*. Torino, 1878. Mosso: *Über die gegenseitigen Beziehungen der Bauch- und Brustathmung*, in Dubois-Reymond's *Archiv für Anatomie und Physiologie*. 1878, p. 441.
3. Mosso: *Über die gegenseitigen Beziehungen der Bauch- und Brustathmung*, in du Bois-Reymond's *Archiv für Anatomie und Physiologie*. 1878, p. 461, §. 10.
4. Ibid.
5. In my previously cited treatise, the translator, Dr. Baron Ungern-Sternberg, expressed the opinion that inspiratory lowering of the thorax was also possible, and indeed must occur each time the contraction of the diaphragm exerts a stronger influence on the position of the thorax than the accessory muscles. He asked me to mention here that he currently considers this assumption to be incorrect, inasmuch as the diaphragm, at least under physiologic conditions, cannot influence the position of the thorax at all.
6. Mosso refers to the English philosopher Herbert Spencer's *Principles of Psychology*, first published in London in 1855. The endnote reference states the correct title.
7. Spencer: *Principes de psychologie*. Paris, 1875. Vol. I, p. 86.

On the Fluctuations of the Cerebral Tracings That Are Controlled by the Movements of the Vessels and of the Heart

§. 7.1

Aside from the pulsations, which stem from the contractions of the heart, and the oscillations, which are controlled by the respiratory movements, there are in the cerebral tracings rises and falls that are in general more significant than the preceding ones and that I have termed **undulations**.[1] In this generic term I have included a whole array of volume variations of the brain, which depend on multiple, altogether heterologous causes.

As much as I would have liked to classify **undulations** into different groups according to their underlying causal factors, I succeeded in determining their origin for only a relatively small series of them. All remaining undulations, the cause of which I was unable to elucidate, I have summed up (as one saw in the preceding chapter) under the general designation "**spontaneous movements of the vessels**." It goes without saying that I use the adjective "**spontaneous**" in its narrowest physiologic sense and mean by this, as I have pointed out elsewhere, that the material cause of the phenomenon, the existence of which must necessarily be assumed, remains unknown to us to the present day. It is left for us to hope that this group will disappear by and by and make room for a more natural classification.

The wave-like undulations of the blood pressure, first observed by Traube on dogs and cats and later extensively studied by Hering and Schiff, represent only a special subcategory of the phenomenon to be discussed here. The spontaneous movements of the vessels, when restricted to an individual bodily province, can produce distinct undulations in the plethysmographic (i.e., the volume) tracing of the same, even when the blood pressure in the great arterial trunks remains unchanged, and hence the so-called wave-like fluctuations of the blood pressure are missing. The basis for the possible incongruence of both phenomena becomes clear when one considers that plethysmographic swings are often a purely local manifestation, whereas fluctuations of blood pressure mostly represent a general phenomenon, the consequences of which extend to the entire circulation. In the next chapter, we will turn to certain observations easily carried out on the rabbit, which demonstrate that the vessels can expand in a specific body region and can generate plethysmographic fluctuations without the blood pressure in the large vascular trunks undergoing a change: it is sufficient that the vessels in another province of the body experience a contraction, the influence of which would have compensated for and eliminated the decrease in pressure that otherwise would have to have occurred.

When the plethysmographic fluctuations correspond exactly to those of the blood pressure so that the diminution in volume of an organ is accompanied by an increase in blood pressure and vice versa, then one may assume that the vascular contraction reflects the cause of the pressure increase and the expansion of the vessels reflects the cause of the pressure decrease in the large vascular trunks. During our investigations, however, we have also confirmed the occurrence of an opposing combination, that is, an augmentation of pressure in the large afferent arterial trunks in the presence of a volume increase of the organ in question (respectively, pressure decrease with diminution of volume).

In such cases, one has to deal with a **passive** volume variation of the organ, in which this variation is induced through the intensified (respectively, diminished) blood flow caused by a rise (or fall) of the blood pressure. This type of action can be observed, for instance, in the brain with increased imaginary activity and with mood changes/emotions, when one sees the rise of the plethysmographic cerebral tracing coincide with a fall of the plethysmographic tracing of the forearm. Since the spastic ischemia of the extremities functions here as the peripheral cause of the general pressure increase in the vascular system and of the volume increase in the brain, we see here within the brain a fluctuation of volume, which we can briefly call **passive**.

Later on, in the rabbit, we will become acquainted with a seemingly analogous but in reality substantially different case: namely, a **decrease of the blood pressure with narrowing** of the external vessels of the ear (therefore necessarily also a volume decrease of the external ear). This case would be identical to the one just discussed if the vascular contraction could be viewed as a result of the pressure decrease and the correspondingly lesser flow of blood to the vessels of the ear. Meanwhile, the direct observation of the process in these vessels forces us to assume that we are not in any way dealing with a passive, secondary contraction, an adaptation to the sparse blood flow, but with an active, primary contraction. And if this is the case, then it begs the question why here the local ischemia of the external ear does not (as in the previous case of the extremities) lead to an increase of pressure in the vascular system, but on the contrary goes hand in hand with a pressure decrease. Since during these experiments the strength and frequency of the heartbeats remained unchanged, we must assume that the

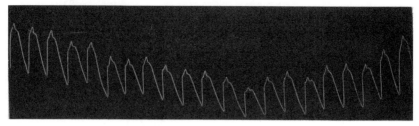

Figure 7.1 Passive plethysmographic undulation of the brain.

contraction of the vessels in and of itself was not sufficient to raise the general blood pressure while there was at the same time in other parts of the body a vascular expansion, which not only cancelled out the influence of the auricular ischemia but also prevailed and thus caused a decrease in the general blood pressure.

In any case, our experiments demonstrate the erroneous nature of the assumption of v. Basch,[2] who relates the swelling of the arm to a rise and the shrinking of the arm to a fall of the aortic pressure.

The plethysmographic variations of the brain that we call passive (which, accordingly, depend on the increase or decrease of the blood pressure without active participation of the specific vessels of the named organ) distinguish themselves from those called active by the variable configuration that the contraction or the relaxation of the vascular walls imparts to the individual pulsations of the brain.

The tracings in Figs. 7.1, 7.2, and 7.3 may suffice to provide an example of this variability.

The cerebral pulse of Bertino was of a definitely tricuspid shape. Suddenly and without demonstrable cause, a fall of the tracing sets in (Fig. 7.1). The individual pulsations decrease in the direction of the abscissa and become smaller; yet their shape remains unchanged. The recording continues without interruption. Slight respiratory oscillations appear in the tracing, which I do not reproduce here, and thereafter (Fig. 7.2) another decrease follows, which varies from the former by a decisive change in the shape of the pulsations: while beforehand these were anacrotic, now they become catacrotic. This change is all the more remarkable as the decrease in cerebral volume is much smaller now than it was previously when the shape of the pulsations had hardly changed at all.

The observations communicated up to now, as well as other facts that we will discuss subsequently, compel us to assume that there existed a primary contraction of the vasculature in Fig. 7.2, while in Fig. 7.1 we must hypothesize first a decrease in blood pressure and then a secondary contraction of the vessels.

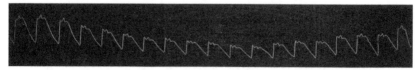

Figure 7.2 Plethysmographic undulation of the brain caused by contraction of the cerebral vessels.

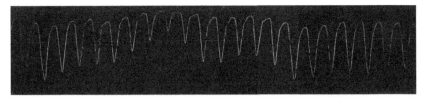

Figure 7.3 Plethysmographic undulation of the brain caused by a variation of blood outflow.

Among the passive plethysmographic fluctuations, we also count those that are dependent on a change of the outflow of venous blood. Evidently, the volume of an organ can increase or decrease when the arterial inflow of blood rises or falls while the venous outflow remains the same. However, volume can also increase or decrease when, in the case of arterial inflow remaining constant, venous outflow is diminished or augmented. If we now consider the tracings of the cerebral pulse, we see that frequent variations occur in the inferior part of the pulse waves, directed toward the abscissa. While earlier on our attention was engaged primarily by the apical portion of the individual pulse waves, we must now direct it to their basal portion.

In tracing Fig. 7.3, recorded with the little Thron, we see indeed that initially the pulsations become gradually smaller even though a slight increase in brain volume takes place, and that later on they increase in height while the brain volume experiences a slight decrease. In the continuation of this tracing, the strongest undulations do not occur in the broken line that connects the apices of the pulse waves, but in the lower line, that connecting the bases of the waves. To explain this phenomenon we must necessarily assume that the first and the subsequent undulations were caused by a decrease of venous outflow.

————————————

During the investigations I conducted about plethysmographic variations, I obtained very similar results to those of Mayer[3] regarding variations of blood pressure. Therefore, I, too, may draw the conclusion "that there is no relationship between the rhythm of innervation for the respiratory movements and that of the innervation for the blood vessels." I will immediately cite an example that demonstrates the accuracy of this statement in the case of man.

Figure 7.4 shows a deep undulation of the brain that developed in Catherina X. during sleep, which does not correspond to any demonstrable external

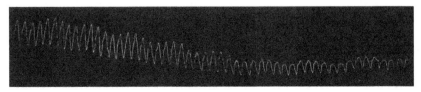

Figure 7.4 Catherina X. A plethysmographic undulation of the brain, which appeared during sleep.

influence and furthermore does not depend on the respiratory movements controlling those smaller oscillations that can also be recognized in the figure. In a similar way, too, one can see in Plate 5.1, tracings 15 and 16, independent of one another, greater undulations of unknown cause and smaller ones controlled by respiratory movements.

There is a phenomenon present here, which has no relationship whatsoever either with innervation or with the movements of the respiratory apparatus (Traube and Hering), a phenomenon that comes about without one's having to posit its dependence upon a venous quality of the arterial blood either due to accumulation of carbon dioxide or to lack of oxygen (Cyon, Hering).[4] For us this is an absolutely normal phenomenon, which we interpret as a change in the elasticity of the vascular walls, because we do not perceive any corresponding modification in the forearm pulse.

There is no constant rhythm to the spontaneous undulations of the cerebral vessels, and since the cerebral tracing may also lack the respiratory swings, it can often remain horizontal for a long time without demonstrating any other elevations than those of the pulse, even when the respiratory oscillations are visible in the forearm.

I have already noted elsewhere that when contour variations of the cerebral pulse and volume changes of the brain which depend on a systemic cause, are to be distinguished from those that are purely local and specific to the brain, the appropriate procedure must consist of the simultaneous recording of the pulse of the brain and that of another body part (e.g., the forearm). Since we have often seen that the variations of the brain and those of the forearm are not correlated, we are entitled to the conclusion that they are independent of each other.

§. 7.2

The observations described previously, conducted on the human subject, have thus demonstrated that undulations of the plethysmographic curve are not controlled by the respiratory movements, and that they are not always in accordance when observed simultaneously on two body parts.

A cursory examination of these recordings is already enough to convince oneself that the undulations are not dependent on a change of the frequency of the heartbeat.

Of interest is the circumstance that at times consecutive undulations of the blood pressure are without change even though the cardiac movements experience very prominent changes. Here is one of the many examples I could cite in support of this.

I recorded the carotid pulse of a dog and for this I used a levered tambour filled with a solution of sodium and sodium bicarbonate. Strong undulations appeared (Fig. 7.5) that were wholly independent of the respiratory movements. The contour of the pulse did not visibly change during these deep undulations dependent on a variation of the blood pressure, while we saw in Fig. 7.2 that much smaller undulations based on vascular contraction, however, were tied to a very conspicuous

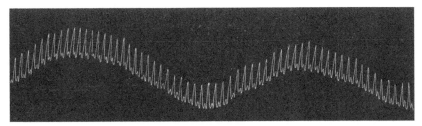

Figure 7.5 Undulations of the blood pressure in the carotid artery of a dog.

change of the pulse contour. In order to see the influence of the slowing of the heartbeat upon the undulations, I exposed on one side the vagus nerve, grasped it with a forceps, and prepared everything for its stimulation by means of an induction current. However, before introducing this, I again applied the pulse-measuring apparatus and waited until respiration had returned to quiet and normal. The undulations continued (Fig. 7.6). At point A, I stimulated the vagus nerve for the first time, and for a few seconds. The cardiac beats slowed down right away, and there followed four or five slower and stronger pulsations. If one imagines drawing a line connecting the peaks of all the pulse waves and another through their dicrotic elevations, one sees that both of these curves continue to rise rather regularly even though the frequency of the heartbeats has greatly diminished. It seemed that a reciprocal compensation between the amplitude and the frequency of the cardiac contractions set in. The median blood pressure value did not decrease by much because the heart, thanks to the much more ample diastole and greater strength of its contractions, and in spite of their lesser frequency, propelled within that unit of time an almost equal amount of blood into the vessels.

At point B, while the tracing was in the process of descending, I stimulated the vagus for a second time, but only momentarily. The contractions slowed down immediately, while the undulation of the tracing proceeded almost without change.

§. 7.3

Until now, we have considered the changes to which the blood circulation in the brain is subjected only in relationship to the activity of the blood vessels. Now

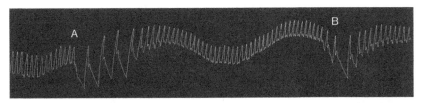

Figure 7.6 Blood pressure undulations in the carotid artery of the same dog during electrical stimulation of the vagus nerve at A and B.

there still remains to be considered those fluctuations of the cerebral tracings that are controlled by the heart.

In the previous chapter (about the blood circulation during mental activity and during sleep), we touched only briefly on the activity of the heart, in order to simplify the object of our examinations and to treat separately the manifestations functioning as factors in this most convoluted process. Meanwhile, there is a constant alternating/reciprocal effect (*Wechselwirkung*) between the functions of the heart and those of the vessels, and if we systematically compare the tracings recorded in the waking state and during sleep, we will recognize this reciprocal relationship always more or less explicitly. Of the numerous examples I could list to this effect I choose only a few, which can be reviewed in Plate 5.5.

In the second half of line 32 and in the first half of line 33, one notices a fall in brain volume, which hinges most likely on the decrease in frequency of the heartbeats; the opposite assumption that the latter phenomenon should rather be seen as a consequence of the contraction of the cerebral vessels (which is the basis for the volume decrease of the brain) appears to be less plausible. The phenomenon occurred when Bertino kept very quiet and there was no external influence known to me acting upon him, while similar changes, visible in lines 34, 35, and 36, had been evidently governed by external stimuli even though Bertino had at the same time been in a deep sleep. In line 34, around the point in time designated by the arrow, I coughed lightly, and there was an immediate decrease in brain volume and a decrease in the frequency of the heartbeats.

At point *T*, tracing 35, Plate 5.5, I lightly touched one of Bertino's ears with a feather. He did not awaken; however, his vessels reacted, as can be seen by the rise of the brain, the pulsations of which became somewhat smaller. Later on the pulsations became larger than previously while the volume of the brain diminished somewhat. At this moment the cardiac contractions were less frequent.

In line 36, while Bertino continued sleeping quietly, a deeper inspiration took place; then, at first, the frequency of the heartbeat rose; however, after 8 or 10 pulsations, there was a very significant drop, soon followed by a decrease of the brain volume.

When the frequency of the heartbeats diminished, one could observe at times a decrease, at other times an increase, in the cerebral volume. We will start by discussing the first eventuality, which I regard as the simpler one.

In the case of little Thron (woodcut, Fig. 7.7), the volume of the brain showed from time to time deep declines that did not correspond to the respiratory movements. While the tracing as a whole descended, the individual pulsations became less frequent and more distinct. I have purposely cited in the first place

Figure 7.7 Plethysmographic undulations of the brain caused by a decrease in the rate of the heartbeats.

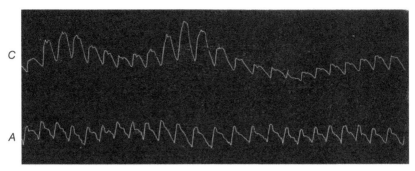

Figure 7.8 Variations of the cerebral pulse *C* and the forearm pulse *A* caused by changes in the state of the vessels and in the strength and frequency of the heartbeats.

the example of a great oscillation, so that it would not appear as though we were dealing with a phenomenon dependent on respiration. At other times the periods of depression were shorter and the individual declines less obvious.

The simplest interpretation of this phenomenon seems to me to be the following. Through the frequency and strength of the cardiac contractions, the brain is kept turgid enough, so that the scar membrane extended over the skull defect can only pulsate very weakly. The venous outflow is not sufficient to shape a significant descent of the tracing at the end of every pulsation (see beginning of Fig. 7.7). Under these conditions the frequency of the cardiac contractions decreases; however, while the pause between them lengthens, venous outflow becomes predominant: this is why the volume of the brain diminishes and the pulsations in the skull breach become more pronounced.

These oscillations created by the decrease in frequency of the heartbeats can recur four or five times per minute, such as we had the frequent opportunity to observe in the little Thron.

In the course of the observations conducted with Bertino during sleep, I listed a few very conspicuous examples of a volume decrease of the brain caused by a decline in the frequency of the heartbeats. Unfortunately, I do not have any tracing in which I simultaneously recorded the respiratory movements in order to demonstrate that during sleep, such variants in the frequency of the heartbeats can also occur when the form and sequence of respiratory movements are unchanged.

In the tracing in Fig. 7.8, the following factors act simultaneously on the cerebral pulse: (1) contraction and relaxation of the forearm vessels, (2) variation of pulse frequency, and (3) variation of the strength of the cardiac contractions. At the start of Fig. 7.8, there are four pulsations during which the cerebral pulse and the forearm pulse undergo a similar change. The sixth pulsation is somewhat shorter than the preceding ones. The volume of the forearm is in the process of increasing, whereas the volume of the brain is decreasing. During the eighth pulsation, there is a noticeable contraction of the forearm vessels during which the volume of the forearm diminishes while the brain volume increases. Thereupon comes a very marked decrease of the pulse frequency during which the cardiac contractions strengthen; however, the height of the pulsations is configured differently in the brain than in the forearm: in the former, it rises significantly at the onset, just when the contraction starts at the forearm vessels, and in contrast it falls subsequently when the forearm pulse begins to rise.

When the volume of the brain experiences an increase due to mechanical causes, as, for instance, under the influence of respiratory movements or with muscle exertion, then a simultaneous decrease in the frequency of the heartbeats does not result in a decline of the cerebral tracing, for the influence of this causal factor is offset by other concomitant phenomena, most especially by the venous congestion.

Relevant examples of a person who stands up or sits down or exerts himself or herself are too self-evident to require at this juncture more extensive discussion of the mechanism of the compensatory effect.

§. 7.4

As concerns the variations that depend on the altered strength of the cardiac contractions while their rate stays constant, I must confess that I approach the discussion of this topic with a certain amount of diffidence, since we are dealing here with a little-researched area of the physiology of circulation, where up until now my investigations on humans and animals have not yet led me to any satisfying result. Even though I must assume that even under normal conditions the strength of cardiac contractions is subject to periodic swings, positive proof thereof, which rests on observation, is still very scant.

To my colleagues who at the bedside find occasion much more frequently to observe significant variations in the force of the heartbeats, I would like to recommend most warmly the strict application of the graphic method and the simultaneous recording of the respiratory movements, the cardiac impulse, and the carotid and the forearm pulse.

If, for the purpose of observation of the pulse, we choose the carotid or another large arterial trunk instead of a more peripheral artery and apply to it a recording apparatus, we often find that even during intense pressure variations the contour of the pulse remains nearly unchanged.

Figure 7.5 provided an example of deep undulations in which the pulse waves only became somewhat smaller during the descending phases of these great fluctuations without, however, changing their type.

After having ascertained the fact that the pressure variations can be very substantial without changing the contour of the pulsations, we will look at another example where the observation was also carried out on the carotid artery of a dog, and where the undulations are smaller but are nevertheless accompanied by much more substantial corresponding variations of the pulse contour.

The contrast with the previous case is particularly striking when one compares a series of pulse waves in the next tracing (Fig. 7.9) and pays attention to the height of the dicrotic elevations. If one imagines a line drawn through the peaks of all the pulsations, one discerns that the tracing fragment reproduced here contains three undulations, of which the first is more pronounced than the two subsequent ones. I have preserved all the tracings I recorded in the course of the entire experiment on this dog while using chloroform, and I found in leafing through them that immediately prior to this use there were much longer periods of oscillation, which were certainly not dependent on respiration.

Sometimes, based on their rhythm, the variations were more frequent and also, along with this, the differences in the profile of individual pulsations more pronounced, as can be seen on the tracing in Fig. 7.10, which was obtained on the carotid artery of a dog of medium size, approximately 2 minutes after injecting him subcutaneously (on one leg) with 0.02 of sulfuric acid of strychnine.

The undulations of the imaginary line connecting the peaks of all the pulsations certainly did not correspond in their contour to the undulations of the inferior line, which connected the bases of the same pulsations (Fig. 7.11).

If we start out from the highest pulsation of every oscillation period, we find that the subsequent ones diminished in height. The pressure decreased during this declining portion of the oscillation period and the dicrotism became more distinct in this process; thereafter followed a seemingly weaker contraction of the heart, without a change in the rate of the heartbeats. The inferior line rose and the second ascending phase of the oscillation period began, in which the height of the pulsations increased again. These oscillations seemed to stem from a variation in the force of the heartbeats.

Their rhythm was inconstant. While at times their duration lasted for barely 3 or 4 seconds, a fluctuation can occur in the same animal and without demonstrable cause, extending up to nearly 30 seconds as one can see in Fig. 7.12, where two short oscillation periods, A and B, were followed by a very long period (C). About 10 seconds later, without there having been a change in the conditions of the experiment, the carotid pulse took on the contour represented in Fig. 7.11, where the periods only encompassed five or six pulsations.

Given such a finding, I naturally wanted to make certain immediately that the phenomenon was not related to respiration. I affixed a pneumograph to the dog and found that the respiratory movements were of the same frequency as the cardiac contractions. I waited a few minutes, and then at the same time I simultaneously recorded the carotid pulse and the respiratory movements. Since I perceived no noticeable periodic change in the contour of the pulsations, I made use of a method already employed earlier and subjected the animal once more to an inhalation of chloroform.

Soon after this, the phenomenon repeated itself; in the tracings, which I have not reproduced in the interest of saving space, one could see that the periodic variations of the pulse contour were not related in any way to the depth of the respiratory movements.

After the chloroform intoxication wore off, the animal again recovered and everything returned to its former state.

I then followed up with a more protracted inhalation of chloroform. Already in the course of this procedure the periodic variations of the pulse again set in.

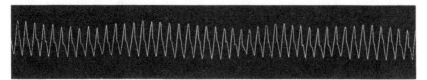

Figure 7.9 Dog. Periodic variations in the contour of the carotid pulse.

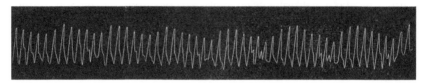

Figure 7.10 Dog. Periodic variations in the contour of the carotid pulse.

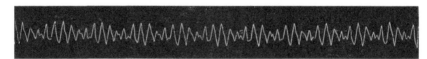

Figure 7.11 Dog. Periodic variations in the contour of the carotid pulse.

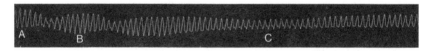

Figure 7.12 Dog. Periodic variations in the contour of the carotid pulse.

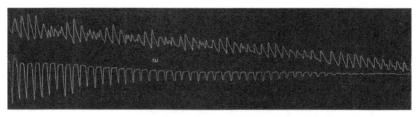

Figure 7.13 Dog. The same under the influence of Chloroform. The lower tracing represents the respiratory movements of the thorax.

At point ω in Fig. 7.13, I motioned for the chloroform inhaler to be removed from the cannula affixed to the trachea.

Tracing 41 permits us to recognize that the blood pressure and the force of the respiratory movements gradually decreased. The cardiac contractions were somewhat more frequent than the respiratory movements, and while the amplitude of the latter decreased in a very regular fashion, the carotid pulse showed very pronounced alternating periods of increasing and decreasing height of the pulsations: periods that lengthened more and more to the extent that the blood pressure decreased.

NOTES

1. Mosso: *Sopra un nuovo metodo per scrivere i movimenti dei vasi sanguigni nell' uomo.* R. Accad. delle scienze di Torino. Vol. XI. 1875.
2. v. Basch: *Die volumetrische Bestimmung des Blutdruckes im Menschen.* Medicin. Jahrbücher. 1876, IV, p. 12.
3. S. Mayer: *Studien zur Physiologie des Herzens u. der Blutgefässe.* Sitzungsberichte der Wiener Academie. 1877, p. 296.
4. Trans.: The German manuscript, which states "Mangel an Kohlenstoff," should read "Mangel an Sauerstoff"; see the corresponding Italian "difetto di ossigeno," which is contextually and physiologically correct.

Concerning the Movements of the Blood Vessels in the External Ear of the Rabbit[1]

§. 8.1

M. Schiff in 1854 was the first to draw attention to the movements exhibited by the blood vessels in the external ear of the rabbit.[2]

As is generally known, there runs in the middle of the auricle, from its base to its tip, an artery, which distributes its branches to both sides, while the venous backflow of this part of the organ is mediated by two venous trunks coursing along its borders. Schiff had noted that the artery exhibits alternating contraction and relaxation movements, which do not correspond to cardiac systole and diastole. If one looks through the auricle against the light, while avoiding any pressure on the vessels, one sees the lumen of the artery narrow periodically and even disappear completely, whereupon the vessel expands quickly again and sends blood into its branches, so that the veins, too, swell up and become larger. This hyperemia of the external ear lasts for a few seconds and gradually fades away, during which time the veins return to a lesser caliber. Schiff noticed such movements succeed each other with an irregular rhythm, most often four or five times per minute, at times rising up to **11** per minute, rarely falling to **two**, and he gave to the artery in question the name of **accessory heart.**

This is not the place for us to engage in a discussion about a name, which perhaps attributes an altogether nonpertinent function to the artery of the external ear. Rather, we simply accept the fact because it has been confirmed by all, but we want to see whether through new investigations we might not succeed in discovering an interpretation of this phenomenon, which parallels or even is identical to the occurrences observed earlier in man, by stripping the vascular movements of the rabbit of any semblance of exceptional significance that they exhibited until now.

In repeating the experiments of my predecessors, I had to take certain precautions, which until now may have seemed superfluous to physiologists. Until now, one had simply conducted these observations by putting the rabbit on a table and holding its ear with one's fingers. Instead, so as to spare the animal emotional distress, I sought to observe its ear in such a manner that it would not become aware of this at all. For this purpose I had a cage built that completely filled up a windowed room and of which one wall, to be facing the interior of the room, was solid so that the rabbits could not see through it. However, into this wall were fashioned a few openings through which I could observe the rabbits in their cage without being noticed. With this simple mechanism I could catch the animals in their usual environment at my discretion and observe them without disturbing their quiet, and without arousing in them the slightest suspicion that one could spy on them. I need hardly note that I fell upon these cautionary measures after I had made the observations described in Chapter 4, from which it followed that the state of the vasculature undergoes very significant changes as a result of external influences heretofore almost completely overlooked.

The observations performed in this manner completely matched my expectations.

The periodic contractions and expansions of the auricular vessels, or in other words, the systole and diastole of the "accessory heart," ceased almost entirely when the animal was at rest. The artery could remain dilated for a very long time, often for hours, without undergoing the slightest contraction. This was especially the case when the animals gave in to deep repose. (I was never able to surprise them during sleep.)

Yet the state of absolute rest was not always accompanied by a dilatation of the vessels. It happened that one observed in the same cage two animals in which the ears of one remained pale for a long time, while in the other, under very similar external conditions, a strong contraction of the arteries came about.

In general, the ears of rabbits were paler on cool autumn mornings than in the respective afternoon hours. Some individuals tended more toward dilatation, others more toward contraction of the ear vessels. Sure, I chose preferentially young and nonpigmented animals (albinos); yet even in old or gray rabbits this same activity can be easily confirmed.

When one observes the movements of the ear vessels of a rabbit at absolute rest, one is almost always able to demonstrate that the cause of the contraction originates in an emotional impression or an external influence. Oftentimes it happens in rabbits that after they have been breathing regularly for a period of time and in the process have retained red ears, a change in the type of respiration occurs: the animal lifts its head and looks about or sniffs, and then a contraction of the vessels sets in and the ears become pale. If all remains quiet, the vessels dilate again after a few seconds. If there is a noise, they contract once more. A cry, a whistle, dogs barking, the bells ringing in a neighboring church, a ray of sunshine penetrating into the cage—all this effects contraction of the vessels when the animal is quiet and when its auricular vessels are dilated.

In this state of rest and quiet, one can recognize that the course of the animal's psychic functions is reflected in the activity of the ear vessels, and that nothing can happen inside the animal or in its environment without it reacting to this with its vessels.

One encounters very often such rabbit specimens with outstanding sensitivity of the vascular system, and I myself had several of them, which through their conspicuous reacting to every outer stimulus have presented not only to me but also to several of my friends a highly interesting and instructive spectacle.

Other specimens reveal almost permanently contracted ear vessels, and thus cool, anemic ears, without my being able to indicate a reason for this.

A pair of rabbits (mother and father) exhibited in this regard an uncommonly stark contrast to its three young. While the latter reacted to all external stimuli with contraction of their ear vessels and at other times showed continuously hyperemic ears, their parents always retained anemic and cold ears.

After I had detected these phenomena after weeks of continued observations of a number of rabbits (10 or 12) and at repeated times, I believe I may consider this as established: that the movements of the blood vessels in the outer ear of rabbits are correlated to the cognitive and sensory impressions and the respective mental state of these animals.

§. 8.2

The changes in the condition of the blood vessels are not the only objectively detectable manifestation through which the swings of the mental state are expressed in the rabbit. If one observes attentively one of these animals in the state of emotional rest, one frequently notices that the contraction of the arteries is accompanied by changes in the rhythm and the depth of the respiratory movements. I have familiarized myself to such an extent with this manifestation that I need only look at the movements of the rabbit's nose to know when a contraction of the ear vessels set in.

After a rabbit had not exhibited any change in the state of the ear vessels for more than half an hour or even only a quarter of an hour, I opened the cage from above, took hold of the animal by the skin of the back or neck, and put it on the table. Seen against the light, the ear almost always appeared pale and anemic at the first moment. Shortly afterward, the artery along with its branches dilated. The hyperemia of the outer ear was so vivid that it did not seem to be less than that which later, in the same animal, set in after transsection of the cervical portion of the sympathetic nerve. The simple visual assessment was sufficient for me to be persuaded that here there was a true tearing apart of the vascular walls, a "**superdilatation**" of the vessels, as Messrs. Dastre and Morat put it.[3] Upon this vivid hyperemia of the ear, a state of pallor first ensued, and then yet another reddening, and so on in alternation, so that pallor and hyperemia at times followed one another up to 10 times per minute; however, under the given circumstances, as a rule only four or five alternations per minute take place.

The animal—and this is understandable considering the fearfulness of the rabbit, which here in Italy is just as proverbial as elsewhere that of his relative, the hare—was completely frightened. Compared to the previous behavior that it exhibited to us in the state of profound relaxation, now its look, its demeanor, its breathing sequence, and the state of its external ear vessels were very much altered. Yet even now, stimulation still succeeded in producing a contraction of the vessels in many, if not most, rabbits. While the vessels were dilating or had already dilated, and while one could presume that they would remain in this state for a few more seconds, one needed only produce a noise, touch the animal, or knock on the table in order to see the ear pale at once. Yet now and then, only in a few rabbits, however, who truly represented an exception, and especially after violent emotional swings, one did not see any contraction of the vessels following sensory stimuli even when those were quite strong, although this still followed very rapidly upon painful stimuli, no matter in which way and in which part of the body those could be brought about. Finally, in a few very rare cases even stimuli of this latter sort were incapable to elicit contraction of the dilated ear vessels: the vessels appeared quasi paralyzed.

If one carefully observes the movements described, I believe one will allow without further question the assumption that the contraction is based on an active process. In the instant when the artery narrows and becomes pale, one often notices individual areas throughout its course, where its diameter is greater, and others where it appears smaller. The same is repeated in the veins, which, here and there, display occasional narrowings, constrictions, and dilatations, which, incidentally, soon fade away.

It was of great interest to determine the relationship that these vascular movements have to the variations of the systemic blood pressure and what controls the contractions and the dilatations of the vessels themselves.

§. 8.3

The arterial expansion of the rabbit's external ear is so marked that one can feel this vessel pulsate underneath the finger. Thus, since one could detect the movements of this artery by mere touch, without visual assistance, it stood to reason that one might in some way be able to chart these local variations of the pulse and compare them to the corresponding variations of the carotid pulse, which is easily recorded in the rabbit.

The first experiments carried out by means of a very light lever, which rested on the auricular artery near the base of the auricle and in its most inferior part, proved very successful.

The animal was free; only its head was held with the hands, which were firmly supported.

The pulse tracing (Fig. 8.1) created according to this process represents the pulse of the arteria mediana at the moment when the ear of the rabbit was strongly hyperemic. Shortly beforehand the pulse of this artery had become so faint so as to disappear almost altogether; suddenly, at point α, we noticed the ear redden and the pulse become stronger and take on the contour reproduced in

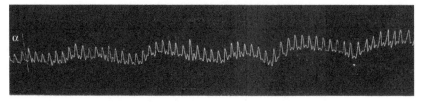

Figure 8.1 Pulse of the *arteria mediana* of the rabbit ear, with respiratory oscillations.

Fig. 8.1. About 30 seconds after the symbol α, the pulse become gradually smaller and disappeared, leaving behind a slightly and irregularly wavy line, in which there was no longer any recognizable trace of the heart rhythm. The respiratory oscillations in Fig. 8.1 were very clearly transmitted, and I ascertained that they truly corresponded to the respiratory movements of the animal, which removed the suspicion that they might be due to the movements of the person holding the rabbit's head.

The experiments I undertook with three rabbits to record the blood pressure in the carotid and that in the outer ear simultaneously did not furnish any satisfactory result. The same animal, on which I had obtained the previous tracing, retained such intensely anemic ears and such protracted contraction of the vessels for more than half an hour after I set it on the Czermak table that I was unable to achieve a pulse tracing.

In this animal, as well as in others, I took all possible precautions to avoid inflicting pain, taking special care to ensure that no drop of sodium carbonate solution entered the neck wound and that any potentially upsetting stimulus was removed; but in spite of all this, the animals' anxiety did not subside, and the dilatation and narrowing of the vessels never showed enough appreciable change to be suitable for graphic representation. I do believe that given appropriate persistence, such an experiment would eventually succeed, but all in all, I did not have sufficient interest in the matter to continue wasting my time with it.

With these animals I restricted myself to examining the relationships between the changing width of the auricular vessels and the blood pressure in the carotid artery.

These observations were not new; indeed, Lovén had already carried out comparable ones in a similar fashion earlier.[4] Yet for the question occupying us here, mine were of greater interest inasmuch as the animals upon which they were conducted had not been poisoned by curare. An assistant recorded the condition of the ear vessels, which I dictated to him, onto the cylinder, right next to the carotid tracing, while I regarded the transilluminated external ear of the animal.

My observations demonstrate that the contraction and relaxation movements of the ear vessels often do not bear any relationship to the simultaneous fluctuations in the carotid blood pressure, although it indeed happens more frequently that a contraction of the auricular artery coincides with an increase, and a dilatation with a decrease, of the carotid blood pressure.

However, Lovén has already shown that in the rabbit a decrease of the blood pressure in the carotid does not always go hand in hand with a dilatation of the artery of the ear.[5]

Since the force of the heartbeats (as could be seen in the tracings not conveyed here) had not undergone any augmentation, one could not assume a general dilatation of the vascular system; therefore, the conclusion had to be drawn that while the arteries expanded in one province of the vascular system, they contracted in another, in order to maintain equilibrium.

After this presentation, which has already been suggested by Lovén and by Sadler (under Ludwig's direction), we must think of the vascular system as being in a process of continuous motion. The alternating contractions and dilatations of the arterial and venous vascular tree have, as an end result, the maintaining of a constant blood pressure. Accordingly, the manometer provides us only one measure for the results of this vascular motion, and if we want to have a clear concept of the circulatory phenomena within an organ, we must take simultaneous recourse to plethysmographic measurements (i.e., to the determination of the volume changes of this organ).

NOTES

1. **Note**: For the sake of brevity I pass over the entire literature relating to this topic and only mention that since the classic observations of Haller and Spallanzani regarding the movements of the mesenteric blood vessels, similar phenomena have been detected in the web vessels of the frog, in the arteries of the torpedo/numbfish, in the tail vasculature of the eel, in the veins of the flying membrane of the bat, and in the vessels of the gills of the olm, *Proteus anguineus*.
2. M. Schiff: *Sur un coeur artériel accessoire dans le lapin*, Comptes rendus. 1854, Vol. 38, p. 508.
3. Dastre et Morat: *Recherches sur l'excitation du sympathique cervical.* Comptes rendus de la Société de Biologie, 1870. The crux of this work performed with the use of the graphic method lies in the determination of the fact that intense and lasting stimulation produces a **superdilatation** of the vessels. However, after a short period of contraction, the paralyzed vessels are capable of a yet stronger dilatation, when the electrical stimulus is powerful and the nerve is sensitive. Dastre and Morat have further shown that the **superdilatation** is not based on the presence of nerves with dilatory effect in the cervical portion of the sympathetic trunk, but on fatigue and exhaustion of the neuromuscular end apparatus.
4. Lovén: *Ueber die Erweiterung von Arterien in Folge einer Nervenerregung.* Bericht d. k. sächs. Gesellsch. D Wissensch. zu Leipzig, p. 85.
5. Ibid, p. 89.

The Influence of Respiratory Movements on the Blood Circulation in the Brain and in the Lungs

§. 9.1

Regular and superficial respiration has such a minor influence on the movements of the brain that it nearly eludes the eye. Only if one carefully examines the sphygmographic tracing of the brain can one recognize that the pulsations decline during inspiration and rise during expiration.

In the recording in Fig. 9.1, tracing *R* represents the respiratory movements registered by means of the Marey pneumograph, tracing *C* the cerebral pulse. Bertino remained perfectly still.

Shortly after, when I motioned to him, he compressed his nostrils with his fingers and remained so for a minute with his mouth shut and holding his breath. Later we will consider the successive transformations undergone by the pulse and by the volume of the brain as a result of such an interruption of the respiratory movements; for now, we will go immediately to the tracing recorded 15 seconds after respiration was restored (Fig. 9.2). In this section, the deep inspirations, which follow a suspension of breath, have stopped already; the pulsations too begin to get smaller. The respiratory movements are somewhat more frequent than they are under normal circumstances. In this case, we see that to each inspiration corresponds a decline in the total tracing, and to each expiration a rise of the same. If expiration lasts somewhat longer than usual, then the decline of the tracing already begins before expiration ends, and becomes stronger with the succeeding inspiration.

The variation of the pulse is all the more substantial the deeper the inspiration is, as one observes in the tracing in Fig. 9.3.

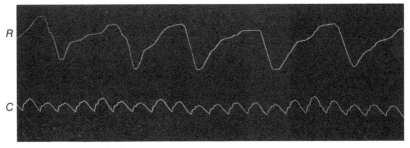

Figure 9.1 Bertino. Influence of normal breathing R on the cerebral pulse C. The respiratory tracing in this as well as in the subsequent three figures is inverted: it sinks with inspiration and rises with expiration.

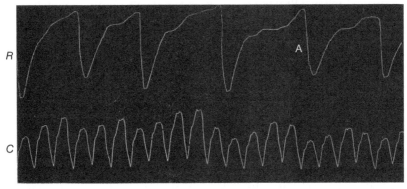

Figure 9.2 Bertino. Influence of a somewhat deeper than normal breath R on the cerebral pulse C.

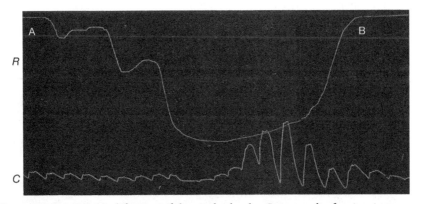

Figure 9.3 Bertino. Modification of the cerebral pulse C as a result of an inspiratory and an expiratory movement, which lasts from A to B.

The experiment was performed half an hour prior to the two preceding ones. While breathing took place quietly and in the same pattern as that in Fig. 9.1, I nodded to Bertino to take a deep breath. I had already explained to him earlier how to slowly expand and compress his thorax. We see that at the end of inspiration, the cerebral pulsations have almost disappeared, and that at the start of expiration they become very ample. I will soon demonstrate that this variation in the height of the pulsations can be explained by the fluctuations of the blood circulation in the lungs, whereby the blood that accumulated in the lungs during inspiration returns again to the general circulation with the subsequent expiration.

I have already demonstrated with an earlier tracing that the volume increase of the brain during intensified mental activity does not rest on a modification of the respiratory movements. Now I want to cite another example, in which one observes two consecutive changes of the cerebral pulse, one stemming from increased mental activity, the other from a deep inspiration (Fig. 9.4).

In the first portion of the tracing, up to the symbol ↓, the respiratory movements present slight irregularities without exerting any influence on the cerebral pulse. At the point where I invited Bertino to multiply 6 by 45, the respiratory movements remain quasi unchanged compared to the variations observed earlier: in spite of this, the amplitude of the pulse and the volume of the brain increase. When Bertino involuntarily took a deeper breath during the mental exercise, the height of the pulse and the brain volume underwent yet another increase. This confirms that the added volume increase of the brain during mental exercise does not depend on a modification of the respiratory movements; additionally, and conversely, it is demonstrated hereby that the swelling of the brain with deep inspirations is not dependent on some psychic effort required for the initiation of such breaths. Indeed, in the present case, Bertino was completely unaware of the change that had taken place in the rhythm of his breathing, as I ascertained immediately after the end of the multiplication.

Between the first increase of the brain and this second one, which was induced by a perturbation of the breathing pattern, there is the fundamental difference that the former coincided with a volume decrease of the forearm, while in the course of a deep inspiration, both brain and forearm experience an augmentation in volume. The observation shown in Fig. 9.5, during which I simultaneously recorded Bertino's cerebral and forearm pulse, may serve to document this.

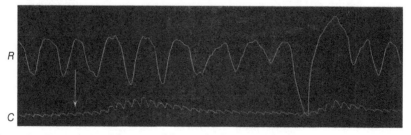

Figure 9.4 Bertino. Modification of the cerebral pulse and volume during a mental operation ↓ and during an involuntary inspiration and expiration.

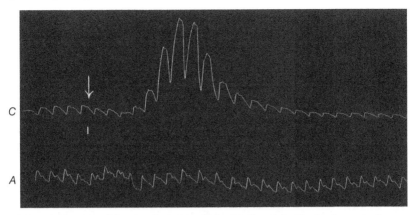

Figure 9.5 Variation of the circulation in the brain *C* and that in the forearm *A* following a deep breath, which began at point *I* ↓.

After I told Bertino about a minute earlier that, after giving him a sign with my hand, he should very quietly carry out a deep inspiration and immediately afterward an equally deep expiration, I inscribed the symbol ↓ onto the rotating cylinder. At the moment when the styli, which inscribe the cerebral and the forearm pulses, arrived at this sign, I nodded to Bertino to begin the deeper inspiration. If we compare lines *C* and *A* of Fig. 9.5, we see that the volume and the amplitude of the pulses both in the brain and in the forearm declined during inspiration and strongly increased during expiration.

A phenomenon that no one, who had carefully studied the tracings heretofore mentioned, could have missed is the greater amplitude of the cerebral pulsations in comparison to those of the forearm. When similar causes are affecting the two body parts, one finds each time the strongest alteration to be that of the pulse of the brain. It seems to me that this fact might be connected with the greater vascularity of this organ and perhaps, too, with the greater pliability of its vascular walls.

§. 9.2

Having procured an antecedent representation of the variations that the cerebral blood flow undergoes under the influence of the respiratory movements, we will now consider a more detailed analysis of these phenomena. Here, I regret to have to declare in advance that the determination of the individual factors that play a role in the variations observed will constitute a difficult task, as is already apparent from the fact that in the interpretation of these factors there have been great differences of opinion between the physiologists who have concerned themselves specifically with these types of studies.

In order to interpret correctly the phenomena observed in the human brain, we must also take into consideration the variations of the circulatory conditions occurring in other parts of the body under the influence of respiration. After finishing the discussion of this portion of the plethysmographic observations, we will subject to an experimental critique the methods and conclusions of several studies most recently published on this topic.

Meanwhile, we will begin with the mechanical causes as being the most simple, and we will try to clarify the way in which pressure variations in the thoracic and the abdominal cavities may modify circulatory conditions within the brain, the upper and lower extremities, and the lungs.

As regards venous outflow, there is not much to be added or subtracted from what Albrecht v. Haller stated in his classic *Elementa physiologiae*:

Magni trunci venosi capitis, abdominis, brachii eiusmodi motu agitantur, in vivis animalibus, ut per expirationem sanguine aut retento, aut a corde refluo turgescant, per inspirationem remisso ad cor sanguine eodem depleantur: hinc per inspirationem, recedente de cerebri magnis vasis sanguine, cerebrum subsidet, idemque eo sanguine per exspirationem retento, et reduce, intumescit et mole crescit.[1]

[Trans.: The great venous trunks of the head, the abdomen, and the arms are, in living animals, agitated by movement in such a way that during expiration they begin to swell up either through blood retained or flowing back from the heart; during inspiration they are emptied of the same blood returned to the heart: hence, during inspiration, with blood receding from the large vessels of the brain, the brain sinks, and similarly, during expiration, through this retained blood it comes back, swells and begins to grow.]

Today, these manifestations, which Haller had detected in the presence of deep respiratory movements, can also be demonstrated with normal breathing by means of the graphic method. The pulse tracing in Fig. 9.6 of the jugular vein, obtained on my sister with the paired recording tambours of Marey, may serve as evidence. My sister lay on her bed and was breathing quietly. A Marey cardiograph applied to her thorax simultaneously recorded the respiratory movements. We see that the level of the jugular vein sinks with each inspiration, for the blood then drains more easily toward the thorax. After the two normal inspirations that one can see at the beginning of Fig. 9.6, I asked my sister to hold her breath for a moment. She held it at the end of inspiration. At this moment, the jugular venous pulse disappeared, only to reappear shortly thereafter and

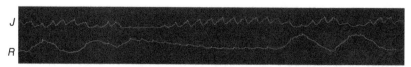

Figure 9.6 Eugenia M. *J:* negative pulse of the jugular vein. *R:* respiratory movements recorded simultaneously with the Marey cardiograph. During inspiration, the tracing *R* rises.

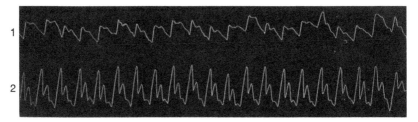

Figure 9.7 Garzena. Modification of the forearm pulse and loss of its respiratory oscillations as a result of increased external pressure on the surface of the forearm.

to strengthen during the subsequent slow expiration. In the interest of conciseness, I will not enter at this juncture into any more detailed reflections on the significance of the jugular venous pulse, having already explained in a previous work[2] that relative to the pulse of the arteries leaving the thorax, it is a negative pulse form.

The same depression that manifests itself during inspiration in my sister's jugular veins can also be detected in the veins of the forearm. I recorded the forearm pulse of Dr. C. Tacconis by means of the hydrosphygmograph, whereby I used such a wide elastic cuff that prior to the experiment we questioned whether it would be capable of blocking the water inside the cylindrical glass container. We took all requisite precautions in order to achieve this and to ensure the success of the experiment from this perspective. Thus, a liberal amount of grease was spread on the skin of the forearm and then the seal was additionally reinforced by pressing the cuff more firmly onto the skin with a circular band applied on top, so that during the necessary manipulations to expel air from the glass container and to fill it with lukewarm water the latter could not escape underneath the cuff. After removal of the elastic band, we noticed that the pulse disappeared. Dr. Tacconis was fasting and his pulse was very weak. We applied two circular loops of the elastic band onto the rubber cuff, and the pulse re-emerged. On this occasion, I noticed an alteration of the pulse, which is of even far greater interest for the question occupying us presently. Indeed, if compression of the forearm veins is minimal, there follows with each inspiration a volume decrease of the extremity; however, if venous compression is stronger and thus impedes venous outflow, the effect of the respiratory movements on the forearm pulse ceases.

In Mr. Garzena, I had likewise observed strong respiratory oscillations of the forearm with quiet respiration (Fig. 9.7); however, when I then exerted a pressure of 20 cm of water onto the entire surface of the forearm, I saw the respiratory variations cease or become totally unnoticeable. To exert this amount of pressure, I attached a vertical glass tube 25 mm in diameter to the anterior opening of the cylindrical glass container of the hydrosphygmograph, and filled this with water up to the 20-cm level. As soon as the pressure stopped, the respiratory oscillations reappeared.

On the basis of these experiments, one might well be allowed to assume a mechanical influence of breathing on the volume of the forearm and propose the hypothesis that with every inspiration, the venous blood flows more easily toward the thoracic cavity and thereby facilitates a volume decrease of the forearm.

§. 9.3

The situation is quite the contrary in the lower extremities: here there is an increase of volume during inspiration and a decrease at the start of expiration.

This divergent activity of the lower extremities in contrast to the upper extremities is easily demonstrated when we undertake the recording of volume oscillations on the leg in the same way as we did for the forearm (along with simultaneous recording of the respiratory movements of the trunk). For this purpose I modified the hydrosphygmograph in such a way as to replace the glass container with a tin boot, which, after insertion of the leg, was filled with water (Fig. 9.8). The apparatus was sealed at the top of the calf with an elastic rubber sleeve or, even better, with glass cement: this way it was easier to affix to it laterally a glass tube *B* of approximately 1 cm in diameter, with which, in connecting the tube to the recording device, we could detect and record the fluctuations of the water level corresponding to the leg pulse and to the other volume changes of the leg. The tin boot and the tube *B* were filled with water from the opening

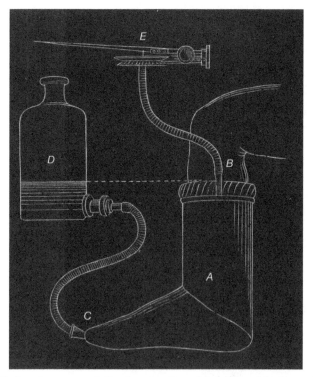

Figure 9.8 Hydrosphygmograph for the recording of the pulse of the lower thigh.

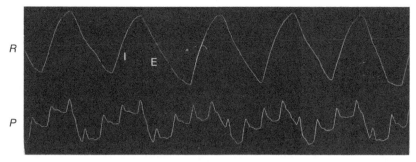

Figure 9.9 Caudana. Volume changes of the lower thigh during normal respiration *R*.

C. The latter was connected to the flask *D*, which can be raised and lowered by a mounted screw so that one can regulate the water level in the tube *B* at will. The levered tambour of Marey *E* served as our recording device.

The tracings in Figs. 9.9 and 9.10 were obtained on Mr. Caudana while he was in a seated position. At the same time as the oscillations in volume of the lower extremity, we recorded the respiratory movements with a Marey cardiograph. The respiratory tracing *R* falls with expiration and rises with inspiration.

The most characteristic fact we note in this tracing is the rapid volume decrease at the start of expiration. Shortly thereafter, while expiration was still ongoing but especially toward its end, the volume of the leg started to increase again. This increase lasted throughout inspiration; at its end the tracing reached its peak, and then suddenly fell with the beginning of expiration.

I asked Mr. Caudana to take deeper and more frequent breaths. The same phenomenon continued (Fig. 9.10). At the moment when expiration began, the leg underwent a rapid decrease in volume.

Accordingly, the antagonism between the plethysmographic tracings of the leg and of the forearm is absolute. For the sake of brevity I will not enter more closely into the mechanical reasons for this contrast. Yet, taking into account that the diaphragm descends during inspiration and that the pressure within the abdominal cavity increases as a result, one might already a priori conclude that during inspiration there occurs a pressure increase in the entire hypodiaphragmatic portion of the venous system. Indeed, such was confirmed by the observations of many physiologists, and only recently by those of Professor Luciani,[3] but to my knowledge no one has attempted to illuminate the effect that the antagonistic activity of the venous outflow in the chest and abdominal cavities must exert on the entire blood circulation.

Since these variations work in opposite directions, their effects cancel each other out, and it follows from their antagonism that the right heart receives the same amount of blood during inspiration and expiration; only during inspiration is the inflow of venous blood through the superior vena cava (thus from the epidiaphragmatic body parts) predominant, while during expiration the inflow is from the hypodiaphragmatic provinces of the body.

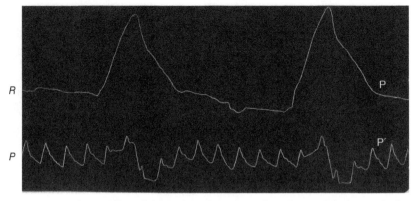

Figure 9.10 Caudana. Effect of deeper breathing *R* on the volume of the lower thigh *P*.

§. 9.4

In my experiments published in 1875,[4] I showed that following deep inspiration the volume of the forearm can decrease by about 6 cm³, and after a series of deep inspirations even by as much as 8 to 10 cm³.

After completing the investigations in question through the study of the changes the cerebral pulse and the brain volume undergo under the influence of deep inspirations, I may now put forth more detail about the causes of this phenomenon.

First, I want to present an experiment I performed with Prof. Fileti in which, using the plethysmograph and hydrosphygmograph simultaneously, I recorded in the same forearm the variations that both volume and pulse of this extremity experience during deep inspiration (Plate 5.1, tracing 20).

In *α↓*, I asked him to take in a deep breath. The plethysmographic tracing *V* descended immediately. The maximum volume decrease recorded by the plethysmograph was 8 cm³. The styli that simultaneously recorded the contours *A* and *V* of tracing 20 (Plate 5.1) were not aligned exactly along the same vertical position as indicated by the orientation points *PP*. In line *A*, one notes the indication of a substantial decrease in volume that the forearm undergoes following deep inspiration, in spite of the compensation of the plethysmograph. The respiratory oscillations, which were hardly noticeable before, became much more distinct after point *α*. The forearm volume returned to its earlier value only after about half a minute.

In the brain, an equally deep inspiration has a much greater effect on the contour of the pulse. So as not to list too many examples, I omit the tracings that indicate ischemia of the brain when there is a series of uncommonly deep inspirations and only mention a tracing recorded with Bertino, in which one sees that a single deep inspiration is enough to elicit a very strong deferred diminution of the height of the pulse (Fig. 9.14, second half).

Bertino remained quiet and immobile. The cerebral pulse was strong and tricuspid, as one can see at the beginning of the figure. At *I*, on my prompting, he took a deep and quick breath. During this, the brain rapidly decreased in volume; the heart rate increased. At the fourth pulsation the pulse had nearly disappeared. With the subsequent expiration *E,* the brain swelled rapidly: the pulse became extremely high. After the end of expiration, there followed a second decrease of the brain volume, this one slower but deeper and more prolonged than the preceding one. The pulse was very small and catacrotic. In other experiments that I performed with Bertino and Catherina X., I saw that after a series of deep inspirations, the cerebral pulse disappeared almost completely.

§. 9.5

Even before my observations of the brain had demonstrated that a strong diminution of cerebral volume, and thus a significant degree of ischemia in this organ, follows after each unusually deep inspiration, it was already long acknowledged that many individuals are incapable of blowing into a fire for longer periods of time without getting dizzy. I could cite the example of an individual in whom two deep inspirations sufficed to induce slight vertigo (Fig. 9.11).

It is then important to determine the manner in which the cerebral anemia occurs. For this purpose, we will first consider the variations that the circulatory conditions in the lungs undergo under the influence of the respiratory movements. In an earlier treatise,[5] indeed, in a chapter where I discussed the movements of the blood vessels in their relationship to respiration, I expressed myself in the following manner:

> Let us assume it were established that, if one artificially brings about a deep inspiration in an extirpated lung, the pulmonary capillaries dilate and the passage of blood through the pulmonary tissue is facilitated: then I hold that the turgor of the pulmonary vessels corresponding to inspiration cannot completely disappear during the subsequent expiration, but that a blood residue must remain, which keep the lungs full and which will disperse only slowly, to the degree that the vessels gradually return to their original volume.

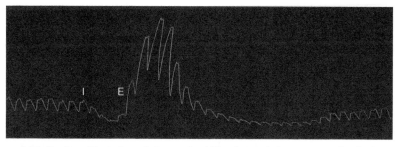

Figure 9.11 Bertino. Variation of the cerebral blood circulation as a result of a deep breath *I E.*

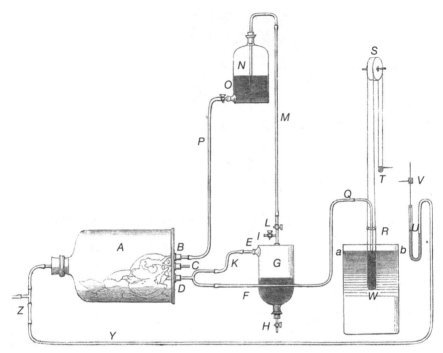

Figure 9.12 Apparatus for determining the difference between the amounts of blood flowing in and out of the lungs during respiratory movements.

I added that I had already devised a procedure in order the question definitively.

This procedure consists of the graphic determination of the differences during the two phases of respiration, between the quantities of blood entering into the lungs and simultaneously flowing out of them, using freshly extirpated lungs with artificially maintained blood circulation and equally artificially effected respiration.

The most important part of the device used for these experiments consisted of a container (G, Fig. 9.12) in which air pressure must remain constant.

One lets the experimental animal bleed to death. Then one extirpates the lungs and puts them immediately into the container A. Using the Mariotte flask N, which one fills with defibrinated blood, one initiates artificial circulation. I omit the description of the less essential portions of the apparatus and of all the manipulations, which are self-evident to anyone more or less familiar with the practical aspects of such experiments concerned with artificial pulmonary circulation; in addition, this topic has already been treated at length by several authors whom I will soon have occasion to mention. I will merely note that the lid of frosted glass through which the cannulae B, C, and D are hermetically pressed was simply set onto the rim of the bell A after covering it with grease. In order to fasten it more securely, I used an elastic band 6 cm wide, which I looped several times around the rim of the bell and the glass lid. This type of seal is much more expeditious than all methods previously used for this purpose and is more than sufficient for the positive and negative pressures coming into question in such experiments (Fig. 9.12).

The blood leaving the pulmonary veins can, after arriving at point D, continue through two thick tubes of equal length: namely, the tube FQ, which leads to the floating cylinder R of the vessel W acting as the plethysmograph, and the tube KE, which empties into the container G. The openings C, D, and E are all at the same height as the fluid level of the floating cylinder R. To save room I will not repeat here the description of my plethysmograph and the way in which it graphically registers the movements of a fluid under constant pressure; for this I refer the reader to my relevant earlier works.[6] I only add for those who might wish to repeat these experiments on the pulmonary circulation that the container G rests on an adjustable frame so that one can easily bring the opening E to the height of the fluid level in the floating cylinder R and the vessel W.[7] That this condition has been accurately implemented one recognizes in the fact that the system of tubes EKFQ is evenly filled with blood, whereby the floater R (into which is plunged the tube FQ) shows no oscillations as long as the artificial circulation is not initiated (i.e., the cannula D sealed).

After the apparatus had been thus set up, I shut the spigot I whereby the connection between the air enclosed in the container G and the exterior air was eliminated, and I opened spigot L. It stands to reason that when, for whatever reason, the pressure in container G decreases, the blood in the floating cylinder must flow into this container. Spigot O of the Mariotte flask N may then be opened to initiate the artificial circulation in the lungs; it is logical that for each quantity of blood leaving the flask N, a corresponding quantity of air from the container G must flow into the flask N.

Here there are three possibilities:

1. The inflow to the lungs is equal to the outflow.

   Since, in this case, as much blood enters the pulmonary artery as exits the pulmonary veins, the pressure in container G stays constant because the amount of blood that flows out of the veins replaces the exact amount of air that comes out of the container and flows into the flask N, there to take the place of the quantum of blood having penetrated into the lungs. The floating cylinder remains still.

2. The inflow into the lungs outweighs the outflow.

   As soon as there is more blood penetrating into the lungs than flowing out at the same time through the pulmonary vein (as we will see occur with inspiration), a negative pressure will tend to set in within the container G. While the pulmonary venous blood flowing into the latter is not sufficient to fill the space created inside by the more abundant displacement of blood from the flask N into the lungs and by the correspondingly more copious flow of air from G to N, the blood in the tube FQ is drawn to the container G and the floating cylinder provides as much blood to that container as is required to maintain a pressure equal to zero within. The tracing drawn by the stylus T records the quantity of blood that has remained accumulated in the lungs in cubic centimeters.

3. The outflow from the lungs is stronger than the inflow (this is a case that, we will see, takes place with expiration).

If more blood flows out of the lungs than is directed to them through the pulmonary artery at the same time, then the pulmonary venous blood, when it has arrived at point D, finds in the tubes two paths of equal width and offering equal resistance. However, at the end of one of these paths is the floating cylinder R, in which the pressure is always equal to zero, whereas the other leads to the sealed container G into which the blood cannot penetrate unless there is compression of the air contained within. One understands that under such circumstances, all the excess blood will pour into the floating cylinder R, and the tracing drawn onto the rotating cylinder by the stylus T will also indicate the speed of drainage of this excess amount of blood from the pulmonary veins.

The expansion of the lungs is accomplished as usual by two glass vessels, which have an opening near the floor and are set up at the same height. The water in the upper vessel, in passing through a rubber tube into the lower, causes by means of the tube ZX a rarefaction of the air in container A. The value of the negative pressure is recorded onto the rotating cylinder by means of a mercury manometer VU, which is connected to the tube YZ. While the lungs are expanding, the air enters freely into the bronchi through the tracheal cannula C, which is open to the exterior.

§. 9.6

Now I would like to describe briefly the course of an experiment. I killed a large dog in order to obtain as much blood as is required to fill the Mariotte flask and to set the apparatus into working order. Then I took another dog of medium size, killed it by exsanguination, and extirpated its lungs, which I enclosed immediately within the container A. After establishing the communications C and D, I opened the spigot O.

The pressure with which the blood entered the lungs was 50 cm. I waited for over a minute to be sure that the artificial circulation was properly under way; then I generated a negative pressure in the container A, the amount of which is recorded by means of the mercury manometer on the blackened paper of the rotating cylinder ab (Fig. 9.13). While the lungs expanded, the stylus of the plethysmograph descended and wrote the line AB, for the floating cylinder R (Fig. 9.12) was emptying, and the blood that was inside streamed into the vessel G to replace the amount of blood that had entered the lungs during inspiration ab and had not exited them. Accordingly, line AB indicated the quantity of blood accumulated in the lungs, and since the floating cylinder was precisely calibrated, it follows that, when we measured the vertical distance of point A from the level of point B, there was present

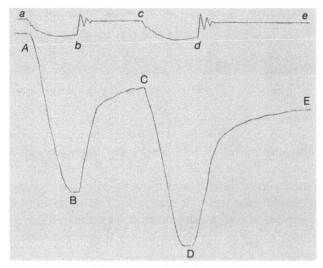

Figure 9.13 Determination of the amount of blood accumulating in the lungs following inspiration.

in the lungs at the end of inspiration an accumulation of 42 cm^3 of excess blood. Next, expiration took place in *bc* (Fig. 9.13) as I reduced the pressure in container *A* to zero by opening the tube *Z* (Fig. 9.12), and as a result of this the lungs collapsed. The blood did not flow out of the lungs as rapidly as it had accumulated there. One could see that the process of emptying was more difficult: to be sure, at first it took place quickly and thus the tracing *BC* rose steeply; later, however, the latter deviated from its original course further to the right and tended to adopt a horizontal direction while there still remained an excess of 15 cm^3 of blood in the lungs. A new inspiration *cd* was carried out, and again an excess of 40 cm^3 of blood collected in the lungs, *CD*. With the expiration *de*, the lungs did not instantly or completely rid themselves of this excess. Even if we protracted the expiration, there remained always an excess of 16 cm^3 of blood that the lungs had not yet thrown off (tracing portion *DE*).

This experiment demonstrates that what takes place in the lungs is the same as what occurs in the skin of the extremities and in all other body parts as is well known to everyone: namely, that when the vessels have dilated under the influence of negative pressure, they fill up with excess blood and after the end of aspiration do not return immediately to their earlier state but need some time to empty.

Even if one wanted to assume that the excess filling of blood could be greater in the extirpated lungs than in the lungs of a living animal, the fact nevertheless remains that following deep inspirations, a certain amount of blood is stored in the lungs that, in the course of the subsequent expirations, is not returned instantaneously to the general circulation, but rather with some hesitation. In order to exclude the complicating circumstance of a rapid change in the elasticity of the vascular walls, I had taken all necessary steps to be able to conduct the

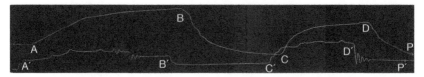

Figure 9.14 Determination of the effect exerted on the pulmonary blood circulation by artificial respiration, brought about by the blowing of air into the airways.

experiment as soon as possible after the death of the animal and felt bound to repeat the experiment not more than two or three times using the same lung.

Having confirmed the factual accumulation of blood during inspiration with the lungs of three animals, I undertook by means of the same device to measure the changes that the pulmonary circulation undergoes when one brings about the artificial respiration with a bellows connected to the trachea.

Since it would have been superfluous during these experiments to place the lungs in the container *A* (Fig. 9.12), I preferred to open the thorax wide, insert a cannula into the right ventricle and another into the left atrium, and then immediately initiate artificial circulation. I need hardly note that for this experiment, as for the previous ones, I had sacrificed a large dog, had filled the Mariotte flask with its blood, and had prepared the recording apparatus so that everything could start operating without delay.

The experiment in question (Fig. 9.14) was performed on a dog of medium size. A wide opening was made in the thorax, and the lungs were left in place. The increase of air pressure within the trachea was simply achieved through blowing with the mouth, and the degree of this rise in pressure was recorded with a mercury manometer onto the rotating cylinder (tracing *A'B'C'D'*). The blood pressure was 40 cm.

The course of the tracing *ABCD* (Fig. 9.15) recorded by the stylus of the plethysmograph shows that with the blowing of air into the trachea, the blood was

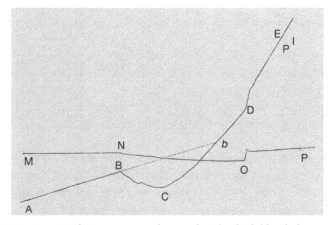

Figure 9.15 Tracing *ABCbDE* represents the speed with which blood, during artificial breathing, flows out of the pulmonary veins during an inspiratory movement (distance *NO* of the manometer tracing *MNOP*).

displaced from the lungs, and that with the subsiding of pressure in the bronchi, the vessels expanded again. One should note especially that the styli were not exactly superimposed, as is indicated by the orientation points *PP* (at right). At *A'*, the pressure in the bronchi increased, as the rise of the manometer tracing *A'B'* reveals. Directly afterward we see that the plethysmographic tracing *AB* gradually rises; that is, there was more blood exiting from the lungs than flowed into the Mariotte flask. The excess flowed into the floating cylinder *R*, which sunk down as a result.

Of interest is the circumstance that here the caliber of the pulmonary vessels increases more during expiration than before, so that what returns to the lungs is not just the same quantity of blood as that displaced during inspiration—an additional surplus of blood penetrates and is accumulated in the pulmonary vessels.

The obvious assumption, which comes to mind here, is that one is dealing simply with an alteration of the vascular tone; however, I prefer for the moment to refrain from taking a position on this question until such time as I have concluded further experiments on the subject.

A second insufflation was performed, and the same manifestations set in again.

We have here, with regard to the quantity of blood remaining in the lungs, a perfect contrast between the natural and the artificial respiration: indeed, we saw that when the lungs, as happens during natural breathing, expand under the influence of negative pressure (i.e., by the lowering of external pressure on their pleural surface [covered by pleura] below that of the free atmospheric pressure acting from the interior via the airways), blood accumulates inside, while on the other hand their blood content diminishes when their expansion is brought about by increasing the air pressure acting from the interior/proximally in the airways.

§. 9.7

Until now we have only taken into consideration the difference between the amount of blood entering into and flowing out of the lungs; the greater or lesser rapidity with which the blood flows in them during the various respiratory phases was not further regarded. With our apparatus, this speed could only be measured visually, according to the faster or slower outflow of blood from the container *G* (where pressure is kept constant).

Meanwhile, we considered it necessary to undertake certain graphic determinations in this direction, not only because such were lacking in physiology until now but also primarily because they are of great import for the critique of both our experiments and those of other researchers.

Where the artificial inspiration was mediated by negative pressure on the pleural surface of the lungs, with respect to the blood circulation in the latter, one must take into consideration the three main sections of the vascular system, the veins, capillaries, and arteries, all of which may undergo expansion. The space created by this expansion was filled up in a twofold manner: once by the copious blood flow from the Mariotte flask, and secondly by the backflow of blood from the pulmonary veins. Since both factors have led to the decrease of pressure in the container G, we need measure only the venous backflow (return) in order to determine the first factor.

I undertook this determination in letting the pulmonary venous blood flow only into the floating cylinder of the plethysmograph. This system allows one to keep the pressure in the pulmonary veins constant and in fact equal to zero, while one has at the same time the opportunity to measure and record the return of blood to the lungs at the moment when the latter expand under the negative pressure exerted onto their pleural surface.

Tracing ABCDE (Fig. 9.15) represents the sequence of an experiment. Each centimeter of the coordinates corresponds to a value of a little more than 2 cm³ of blood. The section of tracing reproduced in the figure encompasses a time frame of 30 seconds. The distance AB indicates the speed with which blood flowed out of the collapsing lungs. Tracing MNOP was recorded simultaneously by means of a mercury manometer. Directly afterward followed a backflow of blood toward the lungs. After the velocity tracing reached its peak at C, it fell with greater speed than it had risen. In fact, if we lengthen the line AB, it intersects with line CD at T: this means that the flow of blood through the lungs has become more abundant.

At the moment of expiration, there was a rapid increase due to the emptying of the veins, and subsequently the outflow continued even more rapidly than earlier, probably because the lungs had discharged the quantity of blood accumulated in the capillaries.

Yet the mechanism of the blood circulation is not at all as simple as we have described it until now. The artificial circulation experiments using a Mariotte flask while the lungs are enclosed in a receptacle replacing the thoracic cavity do not exactly mimic the natural pulmonary circulation of the living animal inasmuch as the pulmonary veins empty outside of the artificial chest cavity and venous blood flows out under the usual atmospheric pressure.

I shall demonstrate in the next chapter that this objection has been given undue weight, for the negative pressure, which starts in the pulmonary cavity during inspiration, is so minimal as long as the airways are unobstructed that one may disregard it. In order to make the critique of this objection more convincing, I shall communicate in the following chapter the results of my experiment about artificial circulation in the lungs with pulmonary blood flowing directly into the artificial chest cavity. And we will see in this case, too, in which all normal conditions are faithfully duplicated, that during the inspiration generated by negative pressure on the pleural surface of the lungs, the blood streams with increased velocity through the lungs, even though the pulmonary venous blood reaches the left atrium under correspondingly negative pressure.

NOTES

1. Haller: *Elementa physiologiae.* Vol. II, Bk. VI. Sect. IV. § IX. 1776.

2. Mosso: *Die Diagnostik des Pulses*. Leipzig, 1879.

3. Luciani: *Delle oscillazioni della pressione intratoracica e intraddominale*. Archivio delle scienze mediche. 1877, fasc. 2 and 3.

4. Mosso: *Sopra un nuovo metodo per scrivere i movimenti dei vasi sanguigni nell' uomo*. 1875, p. 33.

5. Ibid.

6. Ibid, p. 45.

7. In the present drawing, the floating cylinder *R* is filled with blood up to the level *ab* of the fluid located in vessel *W* (a mixture of wine spirit and water). I find this type of arrangement comfortable; however, it is not exactly necessary, as it is enough for the precision of the experiment that the blood level in the floating cylinder, while it fills with blood or empties and thus sinks or rises, remain **constant**, and that the opening *E* be brought exactly to the height of this blood level. If this second condition is also met, then the floating cylinder *R* itself remains immobile, too, as long as the cannula *D* remains sealed.

Experimental Critique of the Investigations on the Pulmonary Circulation Undertaken by Quincke and Pfeiffer, by Funke and Latschenberger, and by Bowditch and Garland

§. 10.1

Quincke and Pfeiffer[1] have established through their experiments about the artificial circulation in extirpated lungs that the effect on the blood circulation in the lungs is quite opposite depending on whether the expansion of the lungs is caused by negative pressure on the pleural side or by positive pressure from the airways; in the first case, the blood circulation is facilitated; in the second, it is made difficult. The results of our experiments cited at the end of the preceding chapter are in accordance with these data. In trying to apply this fact to the natural circulatory conditions, the said authors make the following observations:

> Within the body, the expansion of the lungs is indeed caused by a diminution of the pressure governing the pleural cavity, while the air pressure in the trachea and the bronchi remains (approximately) the same with both inspiration and expiration; however, the pressure weighing on the outer surface of the heart and the great pulmonary vessels also diminishes at the same time and in the same degree as the pleural pressure; thus, if the heart, as we shall for the time being assume for this observation, works with the same force in inspiration and expiration, then the pressure existing in the

branches of the pulmonary artery and vein, relative to the atmospheric pressure in inspiration, will be lesser than during complete expiration; therefore that part of the pulmonary vasculature which is exposed to atmospheric pressure will be less dilated during inspiration than during expiration.

In order to provide a schematic representation of this configuration of the pulmonary vessels and the heart within the chest cavity in relationship to atmospheric pressure, they create the drawing shown in Fig. 10.1. The dotted line represents an elastic tube, in which flows a liquid. The same tube runs freely through the chamber R and hermetically seals off a similar neighboring chamber R'. The chambers R and R' represent two closed cavities that communicate with the outside air only through two superiorly affixed openings. The pressure vessel and the lower container, into which flows the liquid coursing through the elastic tube, are situated in the chamber R representing the chest cavity in which the pulmonary vessels and the heart are enclosed.

The authors state that "with this system, one can achieve with respect to the blood flow through the elastic tube exactly the same variations whether one lowers the pressure to less than that of the atmosphere in the chamber on the right, or whether instead one raises it by the same amount in the left chamber."[2]

From this the authors further deduce that in the course of natural respiration, the blood circulation in the lungs will present the same phenomena as the ones they observed during artificial respiration, when this was accomplished through a rise in airway pressure by means of a bellows.

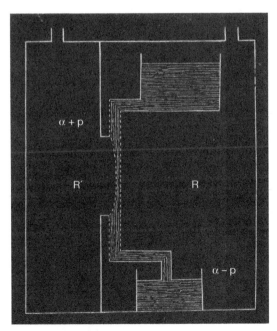

Figure 10.1 Quincke and Pfeiffer's hypothetical apparatus for the duplication of circulatory conditions in the lungs.

Just based on the mere consideration of Fig. 10.1, the matter seems to me to be much more involved than Quincke and Pfeiffer thought. Suspecting they might not have taken into account the fact that the liquid inside the elastic tube is flowing (in flux), I preceded the actual performance of the experiment, which had only been envisioned by these authors, by the following preliminary test. The matter in and of itself deserves more in-depth study, and I will be very pleased if this example of an experimental critique adequately demonstrates the dangers of relying on mere speculation, when in the case of problems regarding the blood circulation there are elastic membranes or tubes being considered. These are factors that carry with them such a motley tangle, and that remove us so far from more accurately researched hydraulic problems, that in this case no one ought to be permitted to venture judgment in a purely speculative fashion without the benefit of direct experiment.

Above all, I wanted to see what would happen with the elastic membrane sealing off the chamber R when the other membrane sealing off the chamber R' is subjected to a positive or a negative pressure, and this while the liquid is in a state of flux.

To duplicate the present schematic representation of Quincke and Pfeiffer (Fig. 10.1), I constructed a small brass box ABCD (Fig. 10.2) in the shape of a rectangular prism, 50 mm long, 25 mm wide, 20 mm high, and supplied with two opposite windows (at C and D), each of which was sealed with a very thin elastic rubber membrane. The small box was further fitted with two oppositely placed, hollow additions (A and B) acting as shafts into each of which was inserted a glass tube 12 mm in internal diameter and 50 cm in length (AF and BK). The tube FA was bent at a right angle and connected with the spigot G of container B via a short and rigid piece of rubber tubing. To conserve a constant water level H, the latter was equipped with a lateral outflow opening L, through which drained the excess inflow of water from the water duct I. The tube GFAK had its outlet at K.

In order to exert alternating positive and negative pressures onto the membrane D, I affixed at the very spot a metallic cupola of somewhat greater diameter than the corresponding window and fastened it hermetically at the lower portion of the small box, as can be seen at D. This cupola corresponds to the chamber R' of Fig. 10.1. So as to be able to augment or diminish the pressure safely and constantly by P, I used two communicating flasks N and M, the latter of which could be moved up or down at P and P' from the level O.

We set the fluid inside tube FABK in motion by opening the spigot G and affixed a writing stylus to the membrane C in order to record its movements. As long as the outer pressure upon the two elastic membranes remained equal to the atmospheric pressure A, a straight horizontal line was traced on the blackened paper of the rotating cylinder. At point A in Fig. 10.3, I exerted on the membrane D a positive pressure +p = 18 cm of water by transposing the flask M from O to P. The membrane carried out an oscillation, during which the stylus recorded the tracing ABCD, whereupon another horizontal span followed at the same level as the preceding one. Observation of the resulting tracing revealed

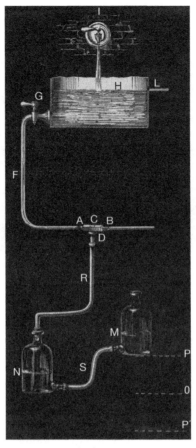

Figure 10.2 Critique of Quincke and Pfeiffer's hypothetical experiment. Apparatus for preliminary testing of the behavior of the membrane sealing off the chamber R' (Fig. 10.1) when that of chamber R is exposed to positive or negative pressure.

that there was a rise B of the membrane, then a fall C of the same below the original level, thereafter a second much slighter oscillation D. The entire phenomenon (i.e., the two oscillations from A to D) took about 1 second. At point E, I returned the flask M to O, which restored the original (atmospheric) pressure a. We then saw the development of two more oscillations of the membrane C; these, however, were in the opposite direction: first the membrane fell toward F, and then it rose and crossed the level G, whereupon it formed a second final oscillation H.

   If we transpose the results of this small experiment onto Quincke and Pfeiffer's schema in Fig. 10.1, it follows that when the fluid in the elastic tube is in the process of flowing or has only one single outlet, then a pressure generated in the chamber R' causes only a momentary oscillation of the membrane D, sealing the other chamber R, but not a continued extension of the same, as one should perhaps expect at first glance. Only the membrane C of the chamber R' undergoes such stretching, and this ongoing extension is expressed by the very fact that when the

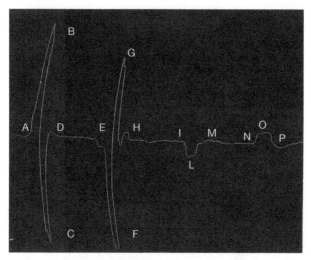

Figure 10.3 Critique of Quincke and Pfeiffer's hypothetical experiment. Tracing of the oscillations of the membrane sealing the chamber R' (Fig. 10.1) in the presence of positive pressure on that of chamber R.

pressure in R' returns to the value A, the return of membrane D to its equilibrium immediately produces a renewed but opposite oscillation EFG of membrane C.

I then performed the opposite experiment. At point I, I exerted a negative pressure –p on membrane D by shifting the flask M from its normal level O inferiorly to P'. To my surprise, the effect was very slight: the tracing recorded the oscillation ILM and then continued again horizontally. At point N, I returned the flask M to point O, and there followed an opposite and very weak oscillation NOP.

Fearing that the difference might perhaps be due to a defect of the apparatus, I closed the opening K and the spigot G at the same time, and while the water in the device was thus still, I found that the pressures a + p and a – p caused a continued tension of the membrane C (in the case of a + p upward, in the case of a – p downward), in both cases much more marked than the rise AB, not to mention the fall ILM, in Fig. 10.3; indeed, the enduring fall of the tracing with the negative pressure a – p was about as prominent as its continued rise with positive pressure.

We dispense with discussing the reason for the different amplitudes with which the membrane C was brought to a temporary oscillation by positive and negative pressures onto D and return to the analysis of Quincke and Pfeiffer's experiment.

§. 10.2

In order to maintain the precise conditions of Quincke and Pfeiffer's hypothetical experiment, I constructed a special apparatus (Fig. 10.6).

The essential part of this device, and the only one that deserves some attention, is the elastic tube inserted between the two containers, in which the air pressure will be as variable as desired (Figs. 10.4 and 10.5; compare also Fig. 10.6, *ABCD*). Here I thought it necessary to alter the layout of the elastic membranes somewhat and I approximated them a little more than in the apparatus represented in Fig. 10.2 in order to counter the objection that the tube experiences an expansion at the site where the elastic membranes are attached. Thus, to build this part of the apparatus, I took a brass tube 13 mm in diameter and 100 mm in length. I cut it lengthwise into two equal parts, *BA* and *B'A'* of Fig. 10.4, and drilled a hole into the middle of each half, through which I stuck a brass tube (*DC'*) approximately 4 cm in length. The two halves were then **sanded** so that they fit together hermetically. I further cut from a thin rubber sheet two pieces about 100 mm long and 15 mm wide, laid them flat alongside each other, and put them between the two longitudinal halves of the brass tube, which I pressed firmly to the adjacent rubber plates with a metal wire wound several times around the entire length of the tube.

These two plates represent the walls of the elastic tube, which was inserted between the two vacuum chambers of Quincke and Pfeiffer's hypothetical apparatus. In order to lengthen the ends of this elastic tube into two rigid tubes, an upper and a lower tube that connect it with the upper and lower vessels, I took two glass tubes 11 mm in diameter, gave them a slightly conical shape by drawing them out over the lamp flame as is represented by the two pieces *F* and *G* of Fig. 10.4, and pushed them between the two elastic membranes.

Figure 10.5 represents a cross-section of the right terminal portion of the system indicated in Fig. 10.4. *A* and *A'* represent the two longitudinal halves of the brass tube, not yet firmly pressed together; *M* and *N* the two elastic membranes; *F* the glass tube.

Since the thickness of the latter amounted to approximately 1 mm, the brass tube was carefully sealed with them at both ends. To be sure that the water would flow between the two rubber plates without penetrating outwardly at their contact rims, I put on a collar of sealing wax and covered the entire tube with a thick varnish. All was now airtight, so that the space between the two elastic membranes (which with the passage of the fluid had to transform itself into the

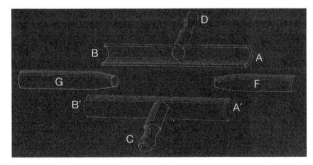

Figure 10.4 Critique of Quincke and Pfeiffer's hypothetical experiment. Device for the reception of the elastic tube.

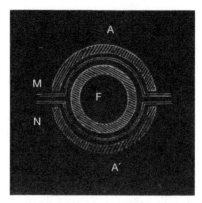

Figure 10.5 Cross-section of the elastic tube composed of rubber plates *M* and *N,* inclusive of the glass tube *F* and the metallic capsule *A A',* corresponding to the right end of the apparatus represented in Fig. 10.4.

opening of an elastic tube), as well as the two lateral chambers, was hermetically closed to the exterior.

Figure 10.6 shows the arrangement of the remaining parts of the apparatus. To the tube *A* I attached a mercury manometer, and I extended the glass tube *EO* to the bottom of the Mariotte flask *G*, which is closed by a spigot *O* (the internal opening/lumen of which is equal in diameter to the tube *E*). Starting from part *B,* I extended the tube *H* into the container *I,* which was fitted with a stopper with two openings: through one of them an extension of the tube *H* was inserted, while the tube *R* came out of the other.

To raise the air pressure in one of the lateral chambers of the brass tube from *a* (atmospheric pressure) to *a* + *p* (as is indicated to the left of Fig. 10.1) during the performance of the experiment envisioned by Quincke and Pfeiffer, the portion of the apparatus just described was sufficient. However, to lower the pressure in one of the chambers from *a* to *a* – *p* (the value indicated in Quincke and Pfeiffer's schematic in Fig. 10.1), another, secondary mechanism had to be set up, which made it possible to put the Mariotte flask, a wall of the elastic tube, and the vessel serving as the receptacle for the outflowing water under the pressure *a* – *p* simultaneously. As can be seen in the figure, this is easily achieved if one connects the openings *Q, D,* and *R* to a glass tube *PST* in which one generates a negative pressure by means of the two vessels *M* and *N*.

In each experiment, I filled the Mariotte flask up to the line I carved into its neck with a diamond. The flask holds 930 cm³. With a watch recording fifths of a second, and which one can start or stop with a simple push of a button, I measured the time in which the flask emptied until the first air bubble passed through the spigot *O*. The length of the tube from *O* to *C* was 35 cm.

§. 10.3

During the experimental examination of Quincke and Pfeiffer's theoretical discussion, I obtained the results recorded in the tables following later.

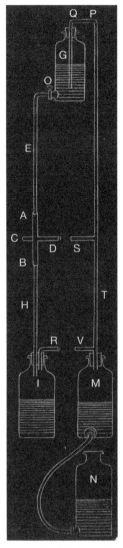

Figure 10.6 Critique of Quincke and Pfeiffer's hypothetical experiment. Organization of the entire apparatus that I used for the actual performance of this experiment.

The first column, with the heading **Normal**, indicates the time in fifths of a second in which the vessel emptied while the openings *PCD* and *R* remained open, or, in other words, while the entire apparatus was under atmospheric pressure. In the second column, with the heading *a* + *p*, one finds the duration in which the vessel *F* emptied while the air in chamber *C*, which was in contact with the outer wall surface of the elastic tube, was under the pressure of a water column of 23 cm. In order to maintain this pressure increase +*p* = 23 cm of water, it was enough to insert the tube *V* into the opening *C* and to raise the receptacle *N* until the water level in this receptacle was 23 cm higher than in *M*. The opening *D* communicates with the outside air. In the last column, *a* − *p*, the entire system was exposed to the negative pressure of 23 cm of water: that is, the vessels *M* and

N communicated by means of the tube *PT* and its lateral portions *V* and *S* with tube *R* and the openings *D* and *Q*. The difference between the water level in *M* and *N* is also 23 cm, but this time the receptacle *N* is the lower one. The opening *C* communicated freely with the outside air.

Part *A* of the following table includes the results of an experimental series in which two somewhat coarse, 1-mm-thick, elastic membranes were used to create the elastic tube. In the second experimental series *B*, I otherwise employed the same device, but the elastic membranes were thinner and more flexible.

	A				B		
Normal	$a + p$	$a - p$		Normal	$a + p$	$a - p$
0.275	1.080	1.260		1.025	1.165	2.004
0.277	1.070	1.261		1.030	1.161	2.008
0.266	1.063	1.279		1.034	1.170	1.296

The premises upon which Quincke and Pfeiffer based their conclusions were thus not validated by the experiment. These quoted numbers show that if one decreases the atmospheric pressure *a* inside the rectangular container (Fig. 10.1) to $a - p$ (that is, if one generates the so-called negative pressure $-p$), there is less liquid flowing through the tube per unity of time than if one raises the pressure *n* in the left container to $a + p$.

The difference in the quantities of liquid flowing out of the tube per unity of time, and therefore also those flowing through it altogether, can only stem from an inequality of the resistances, since the driving force (i.e., the pressure controlling the flow) and the cross-section of the outflow opening remain the same in $a + p$ as in $a—p$, that is to say, in both cases the same as in the case of *a*. The inequality of the resistances, however, can only have been the result of a change in the size and shape of the cross-section in the elastic part of the tube, since this is the only alteration at all in the state of the entire tube that could have been brought forth through either positive or negative pressure upon one or the other wall of its elastic part. I could not establish how the membranes forming the elastic tube were organized in both cases $a + p$ and $a - p$; however, I am certain for this reason that the cross-section had to change.

I outfitted the openings *C* and *D* (Fig. 10.5) with a Marey recording tambour in order to represent graphically the oscillations of the elastic membranes in the case of $a + p$ and $a - p$. It happened that in the latter case $(a - p)$, the oscillations produced were slower and stronger, which, by the way, was already audible to the ear.

Quincke and Pfeiffer in their work underscored an important concept, for they showed in a speculative way that with artificial circulation in the lungs, when the latter are expanded under negative pressure, the amount of blood flowing through them, depending on whether the pulmonary veins are subjected to atmospheric pressure or to the same negative pressure that causes expansion of the lungs, must be different and indeed, in the first case, greater.

I succeeded in confirming this principle/theory with an experiment per-formed with the apparatus described earlier. Indeed, if we generate in D (Fig. 10.6) a negative pressure $a - p$, that is, we subject a wall of the elastic tube to the negative pressure $a - 23$ cm of water $= a - p$ while the remaining system stays under atmospheric pressure (a), one discovers that the same amount of liquid passes through within a shorter time than in all cases considered earlier. This can be seen in the following table C, which constitutes a continuation of table B.

C

Normal	$a + p$	$a - p$	Negative pressure $a - p$ only in D.
1.025	1.165	2.004	0.300
1.030	1.161	2.008	0.298
1.034	1.160	1.296	0.295

The increase of the liquid flowing through is easily understandable if one con-siders that the cross-section of the elastic tube must increase when only a portion of it is subjected to negative pressure.

The question arises to which extent the results of such experiments can be applied to the natural circulatory conditions in the lungs. For my part, I believe that the circumstances are much more complicated here than Quincke and Pfeiffer assumed in their schematic diagram, since the blood vessels of the pul-monary alveoli do not only expand and contract with the movements of breath-ing but also unfold and collapse, as we will see in the following paragraph during our critical discussion of the investigations of two other researchers.

§. 10.4

Funke and Latschenberger[3] have published two treatises to demonstrate that there is a new factor that must be taken into account in the interpretation of the phenomena observed in the pulmonary circulation.

Their investigations rest on the following consideration:

With every expansion of the lungs, whether generated by lowering the pres-sure on the pleural surface of the lungs or by augmentation of the pressure in the airways, there must take place a stretching of the capillary network in question as a result of the increase in surface, and consequently an elongation and nar-rowing of the individual capillary vessels.

This interpretation is hardly new, for Poiseuille had already developed the same in 1855 in his *Recherches sur la respiration*,[4] in which he demonstrated with animal experiments that "insufflation delays the passage of fluids through the pulmonary capillaries."

Poiseuille's interpretation, as well as later on that of Funke and Latschenberger, regarding the delay the blood circulation in the lungs undergoes following a

pressure increase in the airways is based on the assumption that the blood vessels in the pulmonary alveoli are arranged in the same way as the large circles
on the surface of a globe. If this were so, their interpretation might also be on
target. Yet, injected preparations teach us that the course of the vessels winds in
serpentine curves at the surface of the pulmonary alveoli. If we expand the lungs
by negative pressure on their pleural surface, these windings unfold, and, consequently, new tracks can be opened for the passage of blood, which had earlier
been less, or not at all, accessible. It is thus that we believe we must explain the
facilitation/promotion that the pulmonary circulation experiences during normal inspiration. However, if air is blown into the airways, the course of blood is
not impeded because their capillaries would be overly stretched, but because we
exert a positive pressure on their surface, starting from the alveolar cavity, which
must necessarily hinder the passage of blood.

Evidently, Funke and Latschenberger did not properly weigh the contradic-
tion in which their theory stood to the result of the experiments conducted
by Quincke and Pfeiffer (whereby one must not disregard the fact that these
experiments were carried out under conditions that closely approximated
normal circumstances). Indeed, at the end of Funke and Latschenberger's first
work, right after the description of the experiment of artificial respiration by
blowing air into the trachea in the opened thorax, we encounter the following statement: "Furthermore, we do not have the slightest misgiving about
also transferring our explanation to the respiratory blood pressure variations
occurring with natural breathing."[5] We can by no means share this confidence
of the authors, but must rather emphasize that they did not in any way prove
the truth of their conclusion about the natural respiratory conditions.

The total lack of analogy between their artificial respiratory experiments
brought about by blowing air into the trachea was so obvious that the authors
had to retract their conclusion a year later. They published a second treatise[6]
in order to furnish, as they claimed, the direct experimental proof for the
application of their theory to natural breathing (i.e., to the expansion of the
lungs through negative pressure on their pleural surface). Such proof, they
added, appeared to them to have become necessary since observations existed
that permitted the belief in a contrast between the circulatory conditions in
artificial and in natural respiration. It was stated furthermore that Quincke
and Pfeiffer had already sought to demonstrate through precise speculative
argumentation that such a difference in the circulatory conditions of the lungs
existed only when the beginning and endpoint of the artificial bloodstream
were outside of the pleural space and under atmospheric pressure, but that the
passage of blood through the lungs must also be complicated, in the course of
their expansion, by negative pressure onto their pleural surface when all paths
of the pulmonary blood flow, as is the case in the live animal, were enclosed
inside the thorax.

Since Quincke and Pfeiffer had just limited themselves to this one speculative demonstration and had put forth no experimental evidence for their theoretical remarks, Funke and Latschenberger undertook the *experimentum crucis*

during which, as they stated, normal conditions were to be maintained, and they described a system where the start point and endpoint of the artificial circulation (i.e., the pressure receptacle and the container receiving the effluent pulmonary venous blood) communicate with the artificial pleural cavity.

Yet, with this, Quincke and Pfeiffer's theoretical prerequisites were in fact not at all experimentally realized, since the apparatus constructed by Funke and Latschenberger did not at all meet its purpose and their experiments were far from having been executed with sufficient precision to lend a positive value to the results obtained.

The drawing in Fig. 10.7, which we take from Funke and Latschenberger's study, represents their apparatus. The thorax is represented by receptacle A. The pressure, which generates the propelling force of the blood, is created by the weight of the column of blood in receptacle G, from which the blood flows toward the pulmonary artery through the tube F. After its exit HL from the lungs, the pulmonary venous blood passes through the curved tube E, which is drawn vertically here but is placed in a horizontal position during the experiment in order to be able to control the speed of the blood flow in the lungs during the different phases of respiration. This tube, as well as that designated for the flow of air to the receptacle A, is connected to the artificial chest cavity A by the openings 6 and 4.

Inspiration is brought about by means of a Bunsen water pump attached to D. After closing the spigot f, which mediates communication with the outside air, the air in receptacle A is thinned and the lungs expand. Then one reopens the spigot f and the lungs collapse. The authors made no mention of the height of the manometric pressure; however, since they used a Bunsen pump to thin the air, we must assume that the negative pressure had been so significant that any result was hereby made illusory.

In order to move away from the natural conditions as little as possible, as they wanted to do, Funke and Latschenberger should have respected above all the normal relationship between the blood pressure in the right side of the heart and the negative pressure on the pleural surface.

§. 10.5

For my part, I am convinced that the cause of the confusion currently reigning in this field of physiology resides in the very fact that many authors have estimated the negative pressure arising in the pleural cavity during inspiration as too high. There was in these studies, if I may use this expression, a period of decline, and we must turn to the classic work of Donders[7] about the mechanism of respiration and circulation to find a solid clue for the question occupying us.

Donders attached a manometer to the trachea of a cadaver and found inside, upon opening the thorax, an increase in pressure of 30 to 70 mm of water. This is explained by the fact that in the closed thorax, because of the negative pressure existing in the pleural cavity, the elastic fibers of the lungs were expanded beyond

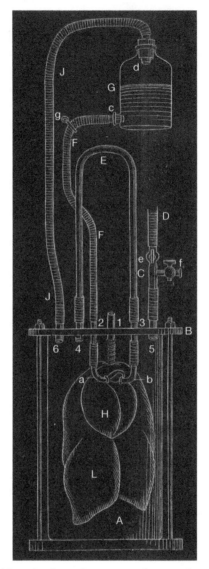

Figure 10.7 Funke and Latschenberger's apparatus for experiments on artificial circulation in the lungs.

their state of equilibrium. If the thorax is opened and the lungs are thus exposed to the atmospheric pressure, the elastic fibers contract by the same amount as that by which they had previously been expanded because of the negative pressure; the narrowing of the pulmonary alveoli and bronchioles occurring in this manner raises the air pressure in the airways by just as much as the arithmetic value of the prior negative pressure in the pleural cavity, the latter of which, in the cadaver, is therefore to be estimated as 30 to 70 mm of water. According to Donders's calculation, when opening the thorax in the live human, there should thus accrue a tracheal pressure of about 100 mm of water or 7.5 mm of mercury, and in consequence this would be the measure of force necessary to expand the lungs so as to fill up the chest cavity, and indeed from the size that the latter has at the end of an expiration. In other words, this is the value of the negative pressure in the pleural cavity at the end of expiration.

However interesting this first determination of the vital resistance of the lungs may be, this constant value of the negative pressure as it exists in vivo at the end of expiration is not critical for our question.

Rather, we should learn what is the pressure required to dilate the lungs from the degree of expansion just considered to the circumference attained at the height of a normal inspiration.

Kramer and Donders have measured in man and in other animals the pressure under which the air flows through the nose and trachea during natural inspiration. Kramer applied a manometer to the side of the trachea of a horse and observed the mercury column of the manometer sink by about 1 mm during inspiration and rise by about 2 or 3 mm during expiration. It follows from Donders's determinations that in the human lung the differences between expiratory and inspiratory air pressures fluctuate between 1 and 3 mm of mercury. The paths by which the air enters into the lungs are so wide, and the resistances to be overcome herewith so slight, that during inspiration the equilibrium between the air pressure in the pulmonary alveoli and the outer atmospheric pressure must establish itself very soon.

It seems to me, therefore, that in patent airways the arithmetic value of the negative pressure in the pleural cavity can hardly exceed 2 mm of mercury. The direct determination of this pressure poses difficulties that to my knowledge have up until now not been overcome. Yet we possess positive data to be able to estimate its probable value under normal conditions (and this is what concerns us above all here). Indeed, since we know that a pressure of about 2 mm of mercury is required for the expansion of the lungs from their circumference at completed expiration to that which they attain at the peak of usual inspiration, that the air penetrates from outside into the trachea under a pressure of approximately 1 mm, and that at the height of inspiration the air pressure in the lungs must equal zero (i.e., equal to the atmospheric pressure), we must conclude that the negative pressure in the pulmonary alveolar cavity during inspiration is almost infinitely small in comparison to the blood pressure in the right heart.

These considerations will hopefully suffice to demonstrate that it was a stark exaggeration on the part of Quincke and Pfeiffer and of Funke and Latschenberger to estimate the negative inspiratory pressure to be as high as they did, and that rather the negative inspiratory pressure should be viewed as infinitely small. The error of their representation will become quite obvious from the analysis of the results of their experiments, to which we shall proceed forthwith.

As we mentioned on p. 128, Quincke and Pfeiffer assumed that the right heart works with equal energy during both phases of respiration. This essential condition was completely ignored during the experiments of Funke and Latschenberger. In fact, if we consider the image of their apparatus (Fig. 10.7), we see that the receptacle *G* from which the defibrinated blood flows out communicates with the receptacle *A* via the tubes *F* and *I*. Had these researchers attached a manometer to tube *F* at the opening 2, as I did, they would have found upon opening the spigot *f* that the blood pressure decreased to a degree corresponding to a negative pressure setting within the receptacle *A*. If one uses a Bunsen pump (at least in the customary way), the negative pressure can suddenly become so significant that its arithmetic value surpasses by a great deal the positive pressure of 40 to maximally 50 cm of water under which the blood must circulate in the lung, and in this case the artificial circulation comes to a standstill. In fact, such was encountered by Funke and Latschenberger, who saw the speed of circulation in the lung decrease after completed inspiration, for they report verbatim the following: "If at the peak of inspiration breathing was halted by the closing of *e*, the acceleration observed during inspiration changed into retardation."[8]

Another failing of Funke and Latschenberger's apparatus is inherent in the method they chose for determining the speed of the pulmonary blood circulation. The idea to attach a horizontal tube that returns to the receptacle *A* after a bend may be a good invention, but it cannot be of practical use for the period of time within which the passage of blood can be observed as too short. One has simply to glance at the picture of the apparatus to be permitted to assert that it was impossible for Funke and Latschenberger to conduct precise experiments, and that their observations must of necessity have been restricted to the phenomena accompanying the first instant of each respiratory phase (*inspirium* and *expirium*).

And indeed, when they tried to repeat Quincke and Pfeiffer's experiments with their device, they were unable to verify what all others have found every time and deemed as essential coincidental phenomena observed at the start of the experiment.[9]

If Funke and Latschenberger could have pursued their observation a little further, they would certainly not have arrived at these contradictory results and would also have found that during inspiration, after the backflow, a more abundant flow of blood immediately sets in, and conversely, during expiration, after a temporary acceleration there ensues an enduring deceleration of outflow, as one can see in the graphic recording of Fig. 9.15.

On the basis of these considerations, Funke and Latschenberger's conclusions regarding the pulmonary circulation seem to us untenable, and we do not consider them in the further development of our topic.

§. 10.6

Much more interesting is Bowditch and Garland's work,[10] especially its second part where the authors report experiments that, even though they were undertaken independently of those of Funke and Latschenberger, were essentially a repetition of theirs and were executed with a largely analogous apparatus. It is true that the authors used the graphic method; however, their apparatus presented the same defect we already underscored in that of Funke and Latschenberger. Indeed, at the moment when the negative pressure is generated in the artificial pleural cavity, the positive pressure in the Mariotte flask decreases by the same amount because the air inside it is simultaneously thinned.

The negative pressure with which both Funke and Latschenberger as well as Bowditch and Garland bring about inspiration would have remained without influence on the pulmonary blood circulation only if the tubes *J* and *F* (we are referring here to Funke and Latschenberger's image) were rigid and if the blood poured directly into the receptacle *A* without first passing through the lungs. However, the container that all the previously mentioned researchers used for their experiments was not airtight, and the lungs, which communicate with the atmospheric air, were inserted into the course of the rigid tubes. Thus, if one generates a negative pressure in *A*, this communicates with the upper portion of the Mariotte vessel and retains the blood within, while at the right opening the aspiration, which should counterbalance this influence and keep the outflow of blood going constantly, is absent. The aspiration coming from the pulmonary veins cannot extend directly to the arterial system, because the entire capillary system, which is in contact with the atmospheric air, lies in between. Therefore, with inspiration carried out in such a manner, the cross-section of the arterial blood conduit must necessarily experience a constraint. If the cited researchers had attached a manometer to the length of the tube *F*, they would have found that at the moment of inspiration the positive pressure decreases by an amount corresponding to the value of the negative pressure at the pulmonary surface.

The first condition postulated by Quincke and Pfeiffer, that for the determination of changes in the state of the pulmonary vessels during inspiration and expiration it is indispensable to maintain a constant pressure under which the blood flows in the right heart, was thus not met either by Funke and Latschenberger or by Bowditch and Garland (all of whom used a Mariotte flask). The mistake arose from the excessive eagerness with which the cited authors were intent on imitating the natural conditions. Just because in reality the heart is enclosed in the thorax, they wanted for this sole reason to withdraw the vessel containing the defibrinated blood from the atmospheric pressure and to connect it to the artificial chest cavity. In doing so, they overlooked the fact that the heart propels the blood into the lungs only through its contractions, not through the weight of the blood. Indeed, one now understands why Bowditch and Garland, when using an artificial heart (i.e., a Mariotte flask in which the blood pressure decreased with each inspiration), really found that during inspiration the blood flowed through the lungs with lesser speed.

§. 10.7

Having established the fact that Funke and Latschenberger's as well as Bowditch and Garland's schematic systems were not suited for the study of the changes taking place in the pulmonary vasculature because their internal pressure did not remain constant, I soon had to contemplate a way to repeat the experiments of these researchers with an apparatus in which the blood pressure in both respiratory phases would always remain unchanged. Even though I had carried out said series of experiments long before Bowditch and Garland's treatise (which appeared in July of 1879) was published, my results are nevertheless applicable without any modification whatsoever for the critique of Funke and Latschenberger's work, as well as Bowditch and Garland's, which had both led to the same conclusions.

The apparatus I used is represented in Fig. 10.8. Taking the precaution indicated on p. 120, I put the lung of a dog into the case A. The defibrinated blood reaches the pulmonary artery from the Mariotte flask G via the tube E and the cannula B and leaves the pulmonary veins via the cannula D.

Into the tube of this cannula is inserted an elastic rubber stopper equipped with two openings. A glass tube runs through the second opening of this stopper to the flask MN, which serves to generate the negative pressure, and the latter is shared via the tube H with the interior of the receptacle A and causes the expansion of the lungs. The same negative pressure can travel/be propagated via the tube PO up to the upper portion of the flask G. The rubber stopper through which pass the venous cannula and the tube leading to the receptacle MN is inserted into the thick neck of a small glass bulb, which forms the end piece of a 200-cm³ graduated burette. The air tube communicates directly with the outside air via the cannula C. This apparatus is based on the same principle as Funke and Latschenberger's work described earlier, but differs from it to the extent that in my system, the negative pressure is not generated by the Bunsen pump but by the vessels M N, and furthermore that it is equipped with a vertical burette for the determination of the speed of outflow from the veins. I determined the duration with a chronometer marking fifths of a second, which was put in motion by pressing on a spring and holding it down. In these experiments, I also deemed it useful first to sacrifice a dog in order to procure the required amount of blood, and only then I killed another to extirpate its lungs and utilize them for the artificial circulation.

In the following experiments, the numbers express the speed of the venous outflow, and this as the time period within which 70 cm³ of blood passes through the lungs; this amount is also assumed in the subsequent experiments. It goes without saying that at the instant when the receptacle N is lowered, a negative pressure originates in the entire system. Since the fluid level in vessel M is 23 cm higher than in N, the manometer K indicates a corresponding negative pressure. The positive pressure recorded by the manometer F for as long as the apparatus stood under atmospheric pressure decreases by 17 mm as soon as the negative pressure of –23 cm has set in within the system.

Experiment I

I killed a large hunting dog/hound and immediately put his lungs into the container A. The pressure, which I shall designate as **normal** (i.e., the height of the

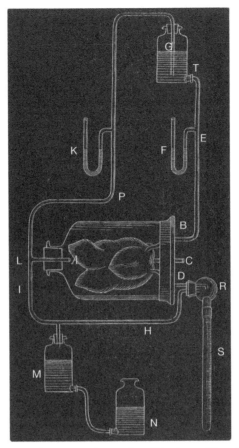

Figure 10.8 My apparatus for testing the results of Funke and Latschenberger's experiment.

column of blood *BT*), amounted to 33 cm. I opened the spigot *T* and let approximately 150 cm³ of blood flow out. Then, to begin, I made three determinations in order to establish the average velocity of the bloodstream and found the following:

70 cm³ of blood flowed out within 0'090
"   "   "   "   " 0'135
"   "   "   "   " 0'145

I generated within the entire system a negative pressure of 18 cm.

70 cm³ of blood flowed out within 0'147.

I lost about 2 minutes because I was mistaken in one of my observations and had to ready anew the vessels *M* and *N* for the generation of a negative pressure of –18 cm in the whole system.

70 cm³ of blood now flowed out within 0'160.

I could make an immediate comparison with the normal pressure because I first had to fill the Mariotte flask with blood.
After about 2 minutes I resumed observation under normal pressure of 33 cm.

70 cm³ flowed out within 1'155.

I created in the whole system a pressure of 18 cm.

70 cm³ flowed out within 1'165.

Immediately afterward I restored normal pressure.

70 cm³ flowed out within 1'166.

I generated a positive pressure of 20 cm in the trachea.

70 cm³ flowed out within 2'281.

Experiment II

The lungs were taken out of a medium-size dog and extirpated immediately after its death and utilized for the experiment. After approximately 200 cm³ of blood under the normal pressure of 33 cm flowed out, I created using the flasks *M* and *N* a negative pressure of –18 cm of water in the entire apparatus.

70 cm³ of blood flowed out within 0'070
"   "   "   " 0'075.

I restored the normal pressure of 33 cm.

70 cm³ of blood flowed out within 0'075
"   "   "   " 0'078.

Negative pressure of –18 cm in the entire apparatus:

70 cm³ of blood flowed out within 0'085.

Negative pressure of –18 cm in the entire apparatus, with the exception of the Mariotte flask:

70 cm³ of blood flowed out in 0'050.

Negative pressure –17 cm in the entire apparatus:

70 cm³ outflow within 0'060.
"   "   "   0'060.

Negative pressure –19 cm in the entire apparatus:

70 cm³ outflow in 0'066.

Normal pressure:

70 cm³ outflow in 0'064.

Negative pressure of –19 cm in the entire system with the exception of the Mariotte flask:

70 cm³ outflow in 0'062.

Negative pressure of –17 cm in the entire apparatus:

70 cm³ outflow in 0'066.

Normal pressure:

70 cm³ outflow in 0'061.

An insurmountable problem that strikes the reviewer of these experimental results is the ever-increasing difficulty of the blood circulation in the extirpated lungs. The alterations produced in these tissues by the artificial circulation progress so rapidly that it becomes impossible to execute in one single animal the entire experimental series necessary for the solution of the question occupying us. Even if one limits the number of normal observations under normal pressure to three to provide an idea of the course of the outflow tracing, during the fourth observation, the speed of outflow, which diminishes continually, can already be decreased by as much as half; soon it becomes so diminished that no further experiment is possible.

In all of this, one may nonetheless conclude with certainty from these observations that in the presence of constant energy of the artificial heart, the velocity of the bloodstream through the lungs during inspiration increases when blood exits from the lungs under negative pressure and flows toward the artificial left atrium R. The concomitant expansion of the pulmonary vasculature is so significant that even when one decreases the pressure in the Mariotte flask by connecting its upper part with the artificial pleural cavity, the outflow velocity stays oftentimes as great as when the pulmonary venous blood flows out under atmospheric pressure. This result can only be explained by an expansion of the pulmonary vessels during inspiration, which counterbalances the deceleration of the bloodstream mediated by the decreased pressure.

If we infer from these experiments a conclusion regarding the natural circu-latory conditions, we hold that **in the course of inspiration, resistances to the passage of blood within the lung diminish.**

§. 10.8

Thus, one sees from these experiments that when one retains the natural con-ditions within the lung during inspiratory movement, a decrease of the resis-tances opposing the passage of blood also takes place. So we have confirmed this according to a different method, which Dr. Aronval sought to demonstrate in his inaugural dissertation of 1877[11] without extirpation of the lungs. In a dog previ-ously bled to death, he compressed the cervical vessels with a Chassaignac écra-seur, opened the abdominal cavity, and introduced into the inferior vena cava a large glass tube, which he allowed to come up to the right atrium, whereupon he fixed the glass tube in its position with a string wrapped around the venous hose between the liver and the diaphragm and fastened it tight. Then he introduced another tube into the descending aorta up to the aortic arch and fastened it in a similar way. After initiation of artificial circulation (with a Mariotte flask), he caused a movement of inspiration by pulling down the diaphragm. The author described the phenomena observed as follows:

> The pleural vacuum increases and an instant later I see the flow through the aortic tube augment considerably. Thus, in inspiration, flow through the lung is easier. If I then imitate the respiratory movements, I see at the moment of the lowering of the diaphragm the blood being called forth with great vigor, and since the valves close incompletely, it is aspirated into the aorta and regresses in the tube. With the diaphragm fixed in inspiration, the flow which had first stopped to allow filling of the pulmonary capillar-ies, recommences anew: I then release the diaphragm which rises in expira-tion, the thoracic vacuum diminishes, the pulmonary vessels themselves decrease in volume, and the blood is propelled by the aorta.[12]

Since Dr. Aronval's unquestionably ingenious observations were, however, performed *en bloc* so to speak, without differentiating between the individ-ual factors of the phenomenon, I thought it preferable to use another process, namely, to extirpate the lungs in order to exclude any interfering influence on the part of the atria, the cardiac chambers, and the great vascular trunks, which were a part of Aronval's experiment.

I had already ended my experiments regarding this when I had the pleasure during a trip to Leiden in 1879 to make the acquaintance of Dr. S. Jager, by whom an inaugural dissertation on the same topic under the direction of Prof. Heynsius had appeared a few months earlier.[13] I spoke to him about the inves-tigations I, too, had undertaken about the blood circulation in the lungs and described to him the process and the apparatuses I had used. I only became acquainted with Dr. Jager's treatise last November, when a German translation appeared in Pflüger's Archiv,[14] and I was thus able to append a reference to this to the Italian manuscript of the present study that at that time had already been submitted to the Accademia dei Lincei in Rome. Thus, although our investigations had been conducted simultaneously and independently of one another, I nonetheless recognize the de facto priority of Dr. Jager in his publication of an experimental critique of this very controversial point of physiology, and I am pleased that both of us have arrived, even though by different ways, at the same results. In spite of this agreement, our two studies each retain their individual character, because each of us had pursued a significantly different process during our experiments.

I also believe that Dr. Jager's valuable work nevertheless has not rendered completely superfluous the publication of my investigations.

In addition to this, during my editing of these pages, a study by Prof. Heger[15] in Brussels has reached me; he has also arrived at the same results although in other ways.

NOTES

1. Quincke and Pfeiffer: *Über den Blutstrom in den Lungen.* Archiv für Anatomie und Physiologie. 1871, p. 98.
2. Ibid, p. 101.
3. Funke and Latschenberger: *Über die Ursachen der respiratorischen Blutdruckschwankungen im Aortensystem.* Pflüger's Archiv 1877, p. 405.
4. The base and the lateral walls of every alveolus contain in their thickness a very abundant network of blood capillaries that respond to the expansion or the retraction of the alveolar cavity in such a way that, given that the surface area of the alveolus increases during inspiration, the capillaries lengthen and their diameter is at the same time diminished. In contrast, during expiration, with regard to the retraction of the alveolus, while its surface diminishes, the diameter of the capillaries increases and their length diminishes. Poiseuille: *Recherches sur la respiration.* Comptes rendus, 1855, Vol. 41, p. 1073.
5. Ibid, p. 428.
6. Pflüger's Archiv. 1878, p. 547.
7. Donders: *Beiträge zum Mechanismus der Respiration und Circulation im gesunden und kranken Zustande,* Zeitschr. f. rat. Med. Vol. III. 1853, p. 287.
8. Ibid, p. 553.
9. "If we deviate from the natural conditions to the extent that we subject beginning and end of the pulmonary flow to atmospheric pressure, as did Quincke and Pfeiffer, the opposite result to that predicted as a consequence of the pressure differential, however, set in: with inspiration the outflow from the lung was delayed, even transformed into a backflow, with expiration it was accelerated" (Ibid, p. 553).

10. The Effect of the Respiratory Movements on the Pulmonary Circulation. *The Journal of Physiology.* Vol. II, No. 2, 1879, p. 91.

11. Dr. Aronval: *Recherches théoriques et expérimentales sur le role de l'élasticité du poumon dans les phénomènes de circulation.* Thèse de Paris, 1877.

12. Ibid, p. 52.

13. S. Jager: *Over de Bloedsbeweging in de longen.* Academisch proefschrift. Leiden, 1879.

14. S. Jager: *Über den Blutstrom in den Lungen.* Pflüger's Archiv, 1879, p. 426.

15. Heger: *Recherches sur la circulation du sang dans les poumons.* Bruxelles, 1880.

Influence of the Respiratory Movements on the Systemic Blood Pressure

§. 11.1

Having considered the changes that are generated by the respiratory movements in the small [Ed.: pulmonary] circulation, we go on to the much more complicated question of the modifications brought about by the same factor in the great [Ed.: systemic] circulation.

I must preface the entrance into this field so rich in valuable works but also in multiple controversies with the note that my relevant observations, which I will report in this chapter, have only been carried out in humans, but I will illuminate them by correlating at the same time some of the most recent researchers' observations collected on man as well as on animals.

In the prominent place amid the classic works of Ludwig and his pupils, I first take the liberty to introduce the following words by Einbrodt,[1] which shall provide us with a firm basis of comparison for the facts observed in other conditions and in different animals to be discussed here:

The blood pressure during inspiration experiences an increase, which takes place gradually but steadily, i.e. every heartbeat encounters a higher tension than the previous one. This rise of the blood pressure, however, does not at the onset coincide exactly with the start of inspiration, but only happens during it—in other words, the highest point of a portion of pulse tracing that corresponds to an entire respiratory movement, does not coincide with the time of inspiration.

In order to provide a more precise representation of these variations, I choose among my graphic tracings one where the course of the carotid blood pressure and of the respiratory movements is in accordance with just this law postulated by Ludwig and Einbrodt.

Pulse tracing and simultaneous blood pressure tracing were obtained with the carotid artery of a dog. For this I used a levered tambour equipped with a resistant membrane and filled with a solution of sodium carbonate. In order to regulate at will the resistance of the elastic membrane of the recording tambour, I affixed a series of elastic rings that, in passing over the aluminum plate lying over the elastic membrane, encompassed the entire tambour, or I wound around the latter an elastic thread so that the blood pressure could not project the membrane of the tambour too intensely. When the blood pressure diminished and the pulse tracing became too little, I removed some of the elastic rings, or I unwound the thread wrapped around the membrane as much as necessary until the desired height of pulsations was reached.

The respiratory tracing was recorded with the Marey pneumograph; the tracing fell with each inspiration. The respiratory movements were wide and regular; inspiration was much more rapid than expiration (Fig. 11.1).

We saw, in fact, just as Ludwig and Einbrodt indicated, that the blood pressure during inspiration underwent a **steady** increase so that each new heartbeat "encounters a higher tension than the preceding one," and we confirmed at the same time that the highest point of a segment of pulse tracing that corresponded to the evolution of a breath did not coincide with the phase of inspiration.

Among the most conspicuous manifestations of this tracing is the marked decrease in cardiac frequency initiated by each expiration, which I observed over the course of approximately a quarter of an hour. This is completely congruent with the data of Ludwig and Einbrodt, according to which the frequency of the heartbeats rises during inspiration and decreases during expiration (Fig. 11.2).

One of the first artifacts I utilized to analyze the reciprocal relationships between the blood pressure and the respiratory movements consisted of the artificial raising or lowering of the blood pressure while the animal was subjected to graphic observation.

I withdrew from the contralateral carotid of the animal a rather significant amount of blood. Since the pulse had become weaker, I diminished somewhat the tension of the elastic membranes of the levered tambour by unwinding the elastic rubber thread wound several times around the membrane and the tambour. After the loss of blood, the relationship of the blood pressure tracing to the respiratory tracing had reversed in comparison to the earlier one: one could now see the blood pressure decrease during inspiration, and during expiration at first rise and later fall. Naturally the type of respiration had also changed somewhat. There was no longer any noticed decrease in frequency of the heartbeats during expiration (Fig. 11.3).

I performed a second withdrawal of blood. Breathing became superficial and somewhat more rapid; otherwise, the same phenomena persisted (Fig. 11.4).

For the third and last time, an additional amount of blood was withdrawn from the carotid. The heart beat so strongly that the pulsations were communicated to the entire chest and abdominal walls. This was therefore also visible in the pneumographic tracing, which had not been the case previously. The wave contour of respiration became smaller and more similar to the normal one. After a minute,

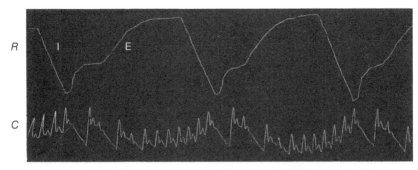

Figure 11.1 Dog. *C*, blood pressure tracing of the carotid, and *R*, tracing of the respiratory movements, recorded simultaneously.

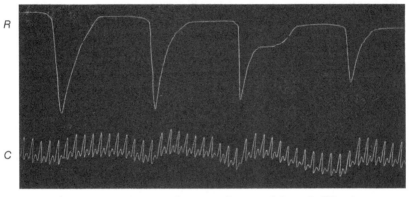

Figure 11.2 The same as in Fig. 11.1 after a significant withdrawal of blood.

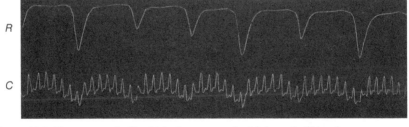

Figure 11.3 The same as in Fig. 11.1 after a second withdrawal of blood.

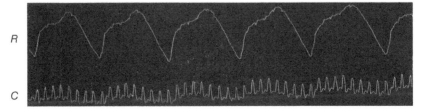

Figure 11.4 The same as in Fig. 11.1 after a third and last (lethal) withdrawal of blood.

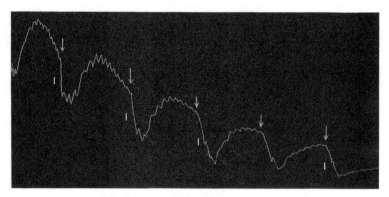

Figure 11.5 Inspiratory fall of the carotid blood pressure after a large bleeding. The points I ↓ correspond to the start of the individual inspirations.

the animal died among forceful and noisy expiratory movements, which were presumably mediated by strong contractions of the abdominal muscles.

With other dogs, the inspiratory decrease of blood pressure during hemorrhage was so marked that it brought to a halt the bleeding from the carotid. Figure 11.5 represents an example of the parallel tracings of respiration and carotid pulse recorded in such animals. In the interest of space, however, I omit the respiratory tracing (the excursions of which were uncommonly great, corresponding to the extraordinary depth of the breathing movements). The letter *I* marks the portion of the tracing corresponding to inspiration, and the upper arrow corresponds to its inception. With the following expiration the tracing rises.

After transsection of the vagus nerves, deep inspirations can lower the blood pressure to zero and make impossible the graphic expression of the carotid pulse, even though the heart in fact continues to beat.

The withdrawal of blood is an effective means to modify at will the rhythm and the contour of the respiratory movements in animals. Furthermore, the greater depth of the respiratory movements in the last two tracings is of no small import, demonstrating clearly the mechanical effect of respiration (Fig. 11.6).

We are dealing here with a purely mechanical causal factor, which enters as a constant in all modifications that the blood pressure undergoes under the influence of the respiratory movements, and which had become increasingly evident through the repeated withdrawals of blood in our experiments.

When the thorax expands, the pulmonary vessels dilate under the negative pressure. If in the course of this the cardiac activity is forceful, then blood inflow

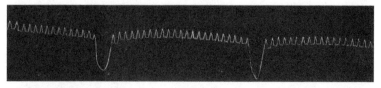

Figure 11.6 Dog after transection of both vagus nerves. Fall of the carotid blood pressure with two deep inspirations.

is so rapid that the space becoming available is filled up immediately; on the contrary, with weak cardiac activity, the same negative pressure can lead to a stoppage of blood flowing in the great arterial trunks of the lungs even though the heart has not stopped beating.

Thus, we are here faced with a mechanical effect, which we must always consider even if it does not manifest itself for other reasons.

§. 11.2

In man, the carotid pulse presents the same modifications as those demonstrated manometrically by Ludwig and Einbrodt on the carotid of the dog.

For example, Fig. 11.7 shows the pulse tracing obtained of my own skin overlying the great left-sided neck vessels, together with the respiratory tracing recorded with the Marey pneumograph at the same time on my thorax. The similarity with the normal carotid and respiration tracing of the dog is perfect, and thus, here, too, Ludwig and Einbrodt's theorem holds: during inspiration the blood pressure experiences a gradual and steady increase so that "each new heartbeat encounters a higher tension than the preceding one." Under the influence of expiration the blood pressure falls, while at the same time the number of pulsations becomes smaller (at least in my case during a prolonged expiration). My tracing in Fig. 11.7 deviates from the Ludwig-Einbrodt principle only in that the tracing C in this instance begins to rise at the exact start of inspiration and reaches its peak at the end of inspiration.

Such graphic images are not new in physiology, since Klemensiewicz already published very similar ones in 1876.[2] Yet what Klemensiewicz considers to be characteristic of respiratory exertion, one can already see in my case with quiet breathing.

The blood pressure increase in the carotid, which dilates the walls of the carotid and causes the baseline of the pulse tracing to rise, would manifest itself even more clearly if the tambour rested only on the carotid. The diminution

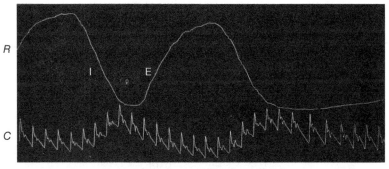

Figure 11.7 A. Mosso. *R,* respiratory movements of the thorax, recorded with a Marey pneumograph. *C,* pulse of the skin covering the great cervical vessels, recorded simultaneously with a Marey tambour applied to the same.

in volume, which the neck veins experience during inspiration, has an opposite effect on the graphic image and thus lessens the effective height of the tracing.

Indeed, if we set the tambour on the median line over the trachea and somewhat above the jugular sternal notch or if we move it above/beyond the veins descending next to the carotid, we see the tracing go down immediately and notice during inspiration a fall instead of a rise (see Fig. 11.8, which behaves in a completely opposite way from the line C in Fig. 11.7).

The inspiratory rise visible over the cervical vessels thus constitutes only the reflection of the difference between the effective expansion of the carotid through increased pressure and the collapse of the neighboring veins.

The same is true also for the forearm. On the one hand, the outflow of blood toward the thorax, made easier during inspiration, must facilitate the emptying not only of the jugular veins and other venous trunks situated closer to the heart but also of the veins in the upper extremities. This factor endeavors to bring about an **inspiratory decrease in volume** in the upper extremities in the same manner as it strives to bring forth at the neck an inspiratory fall of the epidermal covering over the great vessels.

On the other hand, the respiratory and, indeed, the usual inspiratory augmentation of the blood pressure in the aortic system gives rise to a corresponding dilatation of the subclavian artery and its branches and causes a parallel expansion of the carotids. This other influence (which leads, of course, to a respiratory stimulation of the arterial inflow) must conversely strive to cause a mostly inspiratory increase in volume in the upper extremities, as well as a mostly inspiratory lifting of the skin over the great vessels in the neck. Thus, there is also in the upper extremities, as in the neck, an antagonism between the inspiratory acceleration of the venous drainage and that of the arterial inflow, and the forearm tracing, as obtained by us hydrosphygmographically, is but the expression of the difference between both factors. Naturally, it is the predominant influence, which is decisive, and accordingly it would be understandable that during inspiration there could occur in the forearm at times an increase in volume, a decrease in volume, and a lack of any respiratory oscillations in volume.

Nevertheless, the antagonism between the dilatation of the arteries stemming from the aortic arch and the collapse of the veins going to the superior vena cava is only complete when both phenomena are precisely congruent in time, which does not have to be the case everywhere and always, but should rather be seen as a chance exception to the rule—the collapse of the said veins, as an immediate effect of the aspiration exerted by the thorax, must coincide rather precisely with

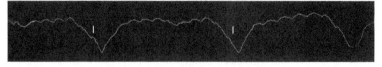

Figure 11.8 Pulse tracing obtained by application of a Marey tambour in the median line of the neck, right over the jugular sternal notch.

the act of inspiration. On the other hand, it is known that the pressure increase in the aortic system, which is the basis for the respiratory dilatation of the arteries, depends mostly on certain conditions controlled by expiration. Among these one must cite above all the circumstance that during expiration, the blood previously accumulated in the lung is returned to the great circulation; then, too, the direct pressure increase that the aorta experiences through the raised expiratory intrathoracic pressure; finally, perhaps also the circumstance that during expiration the right heart (as my investigations have shown) draws blood preferentially from the inferior vena cava, but during inspiration predominantly from the superior vena cava; and that, however, the inferior vena cava represents a much more extensive circulatory area and accordingly has a diameter 1½ to 2 times greater than the superior, which is why during expiration more blood ought to flow to the right heart than during inspiration (on the precondition that the velocity of flow, unknown to us, in the inferior vena cava were not in the same measure less than that in the superior). According to Traube, Ludwig, and others, it is only the arterial contraction, reportedly controlled by the stimulation of the vasomotor center, that acts on the pressure increase in the aortic system during the process of inspiration, precisely near its end. Of the other mentioned factors, the pressure increase due to the direct effect on the aorta of the raised intrathoracic pressure would already assert itself immediately during expiration; the eventual predominance of the influx of blood, coincident with expiration, from the inferior vena cava to the right heart can only prevail after the passage of the affected excess of blood through the lungs. Also, the expiratory relief of the small circulation can influence the arterial blood pressure only subsequently. If one now asks at which point, under the collective influence of these various factors, the respiratory pressure increase in the aortic system must begin, there is nothing very precise that can be stated a priori about this, and we are in this regard solely dependent on **experience** according to which this point in time in fact usually coincides with the phase of inspiration. Yet it is already evident from the start, especially considering the previously mentioned causal factors, that this moment has nothing to do whatsoever with the start of inspiration as such, and can therefore in no way be linked temporally to this. True, Fig. 11.7 reveals that it is not always necessary for the start of the pressure increase to take place only **after** the start of inspiration (as Einbrodt indicates), but that at times it also coincides with this. However, on one hand, the process designated by Einbrodt is to be seen as the most frequent, but on the other hand, we must emphasize that, depending on circumstances, the start of the pressure augmentation in the aortic system, in comparison to its more usual behavior, may be premature or delayed, whereas the inspiratory collapse in the roots of the superior vena cava always remains linked at its onset to the start of inspiration. This circumstance, as well as the changing quantitative relationships between inspiratory acceleration of venous outflow at the origin of the superior vena cava and the (at least partially) simultaneous reinforcement of the arterial influx, provides the next key for understanding the manifold individual and temporal variations presented by the respiratory variations in forearm volume, which extend so far that the volume

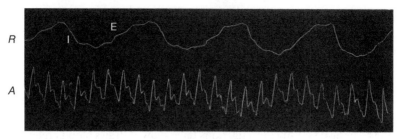

Figure 11.9 A. Mosso. *A*, respiratory oscillations of forearm volume with quiet breathing. *R*, after breakfast.

increase can coincide not only with different stages of inspiration (cf. Figs. 11.9, 11.11, and 11.13) but also with the downright expiratory phase (see Fig. 11.12).

Let us next consider in greater depth a case where the volume increase of the forearm, corresponding to the reaction regarded as typical of the respiratory oscillations of the arterial blood pressure, coincides with the phase of inspiration, and in fact with an early period thereof. This is an experiment that I conducted on myself as a subject and that consisted of the hydrosphygmographic recording of the right forearm pulse together with the simultaneous registration of the respiratory movements of the thorax. The latter was performed by means of a Marey pneumograph. The upper line *R* represents the respiratory tracing of the thorax. During the course of the observation, I remained perfectly still.

At the start of inspiration, the fall of the forearm tracing that had taken place toward the end of the preceding expiration still persisted. During inspiration, this tracing rose. The delay is visibly comparable to the carotid tracings provided earlier. This tracing, too, was obtained in the course of normal, not at all labored, breathing. In doing so, I kept a horizontal position on a table; my forearm rested in a relaxed position inside the cylindrical glass container of the hydrosphygmograph placed horizontally near the trunk and level with the abdomen.

For those who might wish to repeat these observations, I recommend a few precautions, which I cannot deem superfluous, since I see that the experiments undertaken by various colleagues with my plethysmograph and hydrosphygmograph have up to now not furnished the results that I obtained without difficulty.

The elastic rubber sleeve to be fastened around the elbow must be wide enough so as not to hinder venous outflow. I always use a sleeve wide enough so that one can insert the extremity very easily and without effort, which one might even think at first glance is too big. Thereupon I spread grease on the forearm below the elbow, and then I apply the cylinder with its sleeve and fasten the latter around the elbow with a few turns of a rubber tube. As a rule, I wait for 4 to 5 minutes, which I use to place a support pillow under the arm, to set up the horizontal glass cylinder, and to prepare the recording tambours as well as the cylinder of the kymograph. In the meantime, the grease becomes glued to the elastic rubber sleeve, which thus adheres more intimately to the skin. Then I fill the cylinder with lukewarm water, whereby I take care as much as possible to avoid every other motion. After filling the cylinder, I uncoil the elastic rubber tube, the veins empty, water enters from the compensatory flask, and everything is ready for the experiment. The pressure of the sleeve at the elbow is so slight that one cannot feel it at all and that even attentive observation reveals no noticeable swelling of the veins on the forearm enclosed inside the cylinder.

§. 11.3

For such experiments, the times best suited to obtain usable results are the hours following breakfast or lunch. In the morning, on an empty stomach, the experiments almost never succeeded no matter how carefully I proceeded. I really do not know where this discrepancy stems from.

I want to describe here two comparative experiments, one of which I conducted in the fasting state, the other after a meal.

At 8 AM, after having had a cup of coffee around 7, I stretched out on my back in a horizontal position on a table, and I obtained, having observed all the just-mentioned precautions, the hydrosphygmographic tracing in Fig. 11.10.

My assistant informed me that there was no influence of the respiratory movements manifest in the pulse tracing. In order to detect any potential slight traces of such an influence, I had him close the connecting tube leading to the compensation flask.

If one carefully studies the pulse tracing diagonally from the side, one perceives that the respiratory oscillations are not totally absent; however, these are so minimal that with superficial observation they remain completely unnoticed.

Since we are dealing with a negative result, it seems to me superfluous to reproduce a longer portion of the tracing than that provided in Fig. 11.10. Most conspicuous in the part represented here are the strong undulations caused by the instability of the vessels, which are characteristic of pulse tracings in the fasting state. Additionally, I must make note of the fact that the forearm pulsations, which at first glance appear to be very irregular, reveal a rhythmic repetition to their variations, which cannot at all be regarded as accidental or induced by the movements of the trunk and the extremities. Rather, these sinuosities are the

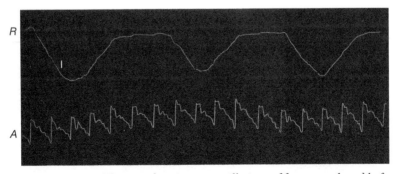

Figure 11.10 A. Mosso. The same [respiratory oscillations of forearm volume] before breakfast.

expression of oscillations that take place in the cylinder and that in my opinion stem from the movement of the blood passing through the vessels, as well as from the impact that each pulsation communicates to the water inside the cylindrical glass receptacle.

Around noon, having eaten a modest meal (a beefsteak, some fruit, a glass of strong wine, and a cup of coffee), I lay down on the table in the same fashion as previously and obtained (using the same rubber sleeve) the pulse tracing in Fig. 11.9, in which the respiratory oscillations are obvious in spite of the lesser depth and amplitude of the respiratory movements. I need not expressly highlight the substantial change of the pulse contour.

To show how much a copious meal contributes to make the respiratory oscillations of the pulse very clearly apparent, I will cite one more observation (Fig. 11.11), which I conducted with my friend Pater D. A. after a copious dinner.

Aside from the much more ample respiratory movements in Fig. 11.11, the course of the tracings is exactly the same as in my own example in Fig. 11.9. We see indeed that the volume decrease of the forearm starts around the end of respiration and continues during the subsequent inspiration. Yet before the inspiratory act is completed, there already appears a very explicit volume increase, which extends into the first period of expiration.

Thus, too, appeared the relationship of the plethysmographic forearm tracings to the respiratory movements in most of my observations. I should be inclined to consider this as the normal type if I had not encountered two subjects who presented, in a state of complete rest and in otherwise similar conditions, different relationships between the volume variations of the forearm and the respiratory movements. An example of such a deviant reaction is the pulse respiration tracing I obtained on Major Garrone, a man of truly giant stature, who kindly made himself available for my experiments (Fig. 11.12).

Here we note during inspiration a volume decrease, which is continued into the start of the subsequent expiration; the increase in volume persists for the entire remainder of expiration. This is a very different, almost opposite type from the previous pulse tracings. The pulse tracing of Major Garrone's forearm

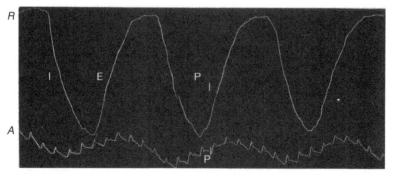

Figure 11.11 Pater D. A. Respiratory oscillations of the forearm volume after a copious meal.

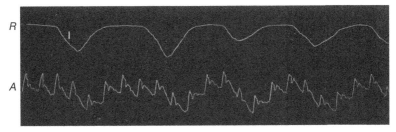

Figure 11.12 Major Garrone. Respiratory oscillations of the forearm volume with quiet breathing.

corresponds to the modification of the radial pulse, which Marey found with obstructed passage of the respiratory pathways.

Having followed Marey, I hoped to arrive at a number of results, which, if I took into consideration various positions, would present the respiratory movements according to the predominant participation of the intercostals or the diaphragm in the expansion of the thorax. I therefore undertook a number of experiments in which I carried out strong diaphragmatic inspirations either with maximum immobility of the ribs or, conversely, where in inspiration I significantly lifted the ribs with minimal participation of the diaphragm; in both cases pulse and volume changes of the forearm were recorded simultaneously. However, in the course of these graphic experiments, which I conducted during the previous fall and mostly using myself as the subject, I unfortunately did not succeed to arrive at somewhat satisfactory results. Rather than enrich the present casuistry by a number of new but unfortunately failed recordings, I prefer to resume my experiments and to continue them as long as necessary for me to succeed in achieving something that will further the interpretation of the aforementioned pulse tracings.

The experiments communicated and discussed until now had been conducted in the setting of regular and quiet breathing, where only now and then at most some breaths might have been deeper, for it is not at all possible for people to maintain the rhythm and depth of their breathing movements completely unchanged when they know they are being observed and their every movement recorded.

Now, however, we want to examine what happens when the breaths are carried out with force and when either the inspirium or the expirium is unusually prolonged.

With Dr. Calozzo, we encounter a different type from that of Major Garrone, for during inspiration there occurs a volume decrease of the forearm, which makes room for an increase in volume even before the end of this phase of respiration.

If inspiration is prolonged, there also follows at first a decrease during the overly great expansion of the thorax, and then a slight increase of the forearm volume.

The volume variations of the forearm are in these cases so marked that it is practical for recording them to use an apparatus, which, as the plethysmograph does, indicates the real value of these volume fluctuations. If such an apparatus is not at hand, it is enough to close the connecting tube between the hydrosphygmograph and the compensation flask in order to gain an idea of the phenomena to be discussed presently.

§. 11.4

If we cast a retrospective glance onto the changes we have seen take place in the volume of the brain and the forearm under the influence of the respiratory movements, the phenomena described in the preceding paragraphs can hardly be reduced to a single norm. In order to arrive at some conclusion, I had to review the entire series of my relevant observations in man (of which I only presented a few in this study). I found that while in the majority of cases the brain undergoes a decrease in volume during inspiration and an increase during expiration (as in Fig. 9.1), and while the forearm mostly begins to show an increase in volume already before the end of inspiration and a decrease in volume before the end of expiration (as in Figs. 11.9, 11.11, and 11.13), there are multiple exceptions. The difficulty in formulating a specific law for these phenomena stems from the fact that here there is a long series of insufficiently known factors so tightly linked together that at times it often becomes impossible to consider in isolation their effects that frequently cancel each other out even under physiologic conditions.

Thus, we see in fact that there exists a diametric opposition between the respiratory fluctuations in volume of the epidiaphragmatic and hypodiaphragmatic body parts, for the heart during inspiration receives more blood from the superior vena cava than from the inferior, and the converse takes place during expiration. The eventual compensation, which may perhaps regulate and maintain constant the influx of blood to the right heart in the course of normal

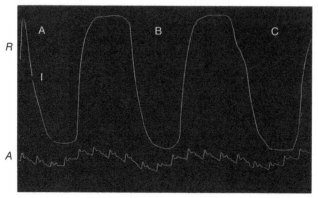

Figure 11.13 Dr. Calozzo. The same [respiratory oscillations of the forearm volume] with deep breathing.

continuation of both respiratory phases, stops in any case under certain circumstances. Thus, there is already a cancellation of the equilibrium in the physiologic width, when the blood accumulates in one part of the body, as, for instance, in the abdominal organs after a meal, during digestion. Since in this case both the influx of blood to the abdominal organs and the efflux of blood via the hepatic veins is augmented, but, on the other hand, as we have seen, the influx of blood from the inferior vena cava to the heart takes place predominantly during expiration, the total amount of blood flowing to the heart during expiration just after a meal must gain the upper hand, even more than might be perhaps otherwise the case (see §. 11.2), over the quantity of blood flowing toward it during inspiration (predominantly from the superior vena cava). In accordance with this, the left heart consecutively will also send more blood into the arteries than during inspiration, which is also why the respiratory fluctuations in all organs (including the forearm) become more marked, as is confirmed by our observations cited earlier. But moreover, the notorious accumulation of blood taking place in the abdominal organs during digestion leads to a relative ischemia of both the lungs and the remaining body regions, which sets for the small circulation conditions similar to those existing after blood losses, when we saw the respiratory pressure fluctuations in our experiments become stronger. This, during digestion, has provided an additional, second, reason for the strengthening of the respiratory volume oscillations.

With regard to the mechanism touched on last, the strengthening of the respiratory blood pressure and volume oscillations is here easily understandable, if one considers that these oscillations rest for the most part on the very fact that during inspiration, the dilated pulmonary vessels fill up with blood more strongly at the necessary expense of the vessels of the great circulation, thus withdrawing blood from those vessels, yet the withdrawal must bring forth an all-the-more visible effect—an all-the-more marked difference in the degree of filling of the body vasculature—the smaller the amount of blood contained within these is.

Of course, one could raise the objection that the inspiratory expansion of the pulmonary vessels need not result obligatorily in a diminution of the blood pressure and the amount of blood in the vasculature of the large circulation, because it is compensated by the decrease of resistances in the pulmonary blood vessels and by the thus induced acceleration of the small circulation. On the other hand, however, it must be emphasized that such compensation does not take place because the resistances in the small circulation generally are extremely small, and that therefore their decrease constitutes a far too insignificant factor for a very substantial inspiratory expansion of the pulmonary vessels for it to be able to conceal and cancel the effect of this vascular expansion.

During these observations, we have postulated that the heart functions with equal strength and accomplishes the same in both phases of respiration. Yet we know not only that the frequency of the heartbeats alternates in the course of the respiratory cycle, and indeed becomes greater during inspiration, but also that the output of the individual cardiac contractions is subjected to respiratory fluctuations that are no less important. The negative pressure establishing itself within the thorax during systole poses a hindrance for the systole of the heart while favoring diastole; the augmentation of intrathoracic pressure that takes place during expiration works in the opposite way. Here there evidently exists an antagonism between the changing frequency of the heartbeats and the changing performance of the individual cardiac contractions, in that the inspiratory increase of frequency must exert an influence opposed to that of the simultaneous obstruction to cardiac systole, and in the same way, the expiratory decrease in frequency in its effects is diametrically opposed to the expiratory facilitation of cardiac systole. However, as regards the influence of the respiratory fluctuations of the intrathoracic pressure on each of the two phases of the cardiac cycle, it must be noted that diastole must be obstructed by the expiratory pressure increase disproportionately more so than systole by the inspiratory pressure decrease.

The study of these phenomena occupying us is complicated even more by the fact that we have no precise knowledge of the influence exerted on the state of the vascular walls by the changed chemical composition of the blood following the respiratory phases, and especially by its changing gas content.

My experiments on the brain and the forearm have demonstrated that deep inspiration is followed by a contraction of the vessels and a volume decrease of the said organs, both too enduring to be explained by the sole accumulation of blood in the lungs. Since this phenomenon is also observed when deep inspiration occurs entirely involuntarily, it is evidently not caused by an effort of will initiating the deep inspiration; rather, I presume that it may be caused by the changed blood mixture without, however, denying that conditions of involuntary innervation could be at play here.

Nevertheless, a decisive judgment regarding the possibility last touched on cannot at this time be pronounced, just as in general the interrelationships between the respiratory and the vasomotor nervous centers are still poorly elucidated.

I pass over those variations of the respiratory oscillations of the blood pressure that can depend on the position of the body and will only indicate that for the phenomenon in question, it cannot be indifferent whether the body assumes a vertical or sitting or horizontal position.

Not without significance here are certainly also the variations that, according to my observations, occur in the state of the vascular walls under the influence of food intake, temperature, and intellectual, sensory, or emotional activity; however, there are still insufficient experiences at hand regarding their closer relationship to the respiratory fluctuations of the blood pressure.

Since all of the factors specified influence the result of our observations, one would have to first research every single one of them individually and in greater depth as to its mechanism of action in order to be able to determine precisely the conditions of the observation or of the experiment in each given case.

As long as the mechanical, chemical, and nervous factors are not strictly separated, we will strive in vain to elaborate the principles of such a complex process.

NOTES

1. Einbrodt: *Über den Einfluss der Athembewegungen auf Herzschlag und Blutdruck.* Moleschott's Untersuchungen, Vol. VII, 1860, p. 314.
2. Klemensiewicz: *Über den Einfluss der Athembewegungen auf die Form der Pulscurven beim Menschen.* Wiener Akademie, 1877, Vol. 1, xxiv, p. 487.

Influence of Amyl Nitrite on the Blood Circulation in the Brain

§. 12.1

Of all the substances known to us, amyl nitrite most powerfully modifies the state of the blood vessels as well as the force and frequency of the cardiac contractions without thereby affecting consciousness or otherwise impairing the cerebral functions in the least. The great facility with which this substance can be ingested, its agreeable odor, and the transience of its effect result in its finding very easy use in our investigations, especially when one has to do with a subject such as Bertino, whose suspiciousness went so far that he absolutely refused to take any medicinal substance if I did not first try it out on myself.

It is known to anyone who has ever inhaled amyl nitrite that a few seconds after the inhalation one feels, as it were, a warm breath suffuse the entire face: cheeks, forehead, eyes, and the entire head redden because of vascular dilatation. Secretion of tears becomes more profuse and one feels a seizing of the head and a sense of anxiety, which is caused by the more frequent and strengthened contractions of the heart.

The process, with which I have measured and recorded the variations of brain volume without distorting too much the contour of the pulsations, has been described in Chapter 2. It consists of the use of two Müllerian valves (Fig. 2.1) that are connected to the tube running from the skull defect to the recording tambour. This highly simple system provides the advantage that the pressure inside the apparatus is kept constant and indeed minimal, while at the same time, through the recording of every air bubble leaving the apparatus or penetrating into it, one is able to measure and register the true increase or decrease of cerebral pressure.

The experiment in Plate 5.5, lines 39, 40, 41, and 42, which I present as typical, was conducted half an hour after a light breakfast, during which Bertino had consumed meat, soup, and bread. The cerebral pulse was small, yet, as one sees at the start of line 39, regular and uniform. In $\alpha\downarrow$, I put in front of Bertino's nostrils a kerchief/cloth upon which I had previously poured a few drops of amyl nitrite.

The man had been instructed to breathe very quietly so as not to change the type of respiration. It was probably the 10th time that he repeated such inhalations, and he understood already very well how to behave in this process. The cerebral pulse tracing continues for a certain distance (about 12 pulsations) without any change. Then, by and by, the pulsations strengthen while the brain volume increases significantly. The elevation S disappears while the dicrotic after-beat becomes stronger. From time to time an air bubble escapes from the Müllerian valve D (woodcut, Fig. 2.1), which distorts somewhat the pulsation recorded at the same moment. At ω, line 39, when the face appeared to be intensely flushed, the inhalation is interrupted. The effect of amyl nitrite persists. A few more individual air bubbles escape from the valve D; the cerebral volume then begins to decrease at M (line 40). The brain pulse still remains very strong. Deep undulations of the brain volume, which do not correspond to the respiratory movements, become noticeable at irregular intervals. More than a minute after the interruption of the inhalation, the effect of amyl nitrite has not yet ended, as can be seen at the start of line 41. From here on the pulse tracing shows fewer high undulations and more that are drawn out in length. The pulsations become gradually smaller and little by little revert to their original contour. The recording continues. At the onset of the second quarter of line 42, already all effect seems to have ended; however, near the final portion of the third quarter at r, a last slight undulation becomes apparent, before the cerebral pulse, and then, about 3 minutes after terminated inhalation, subsides definitively. The recording was continued for another 5 minutes without revealing anything worthy of note. It followed from the number of air bubbles escaped from the Müllerian valve and from the direct measurement of the total volume of an equal number of air bubbles, which I collected under similar pressure in a closed graduated glass tube, that in this case the cerebral volume had undergone an increase of approximately 3 cm^3.

§. 12.2

Let us now seek to clarify the cause of this variation of the cerebral pulse.

As we have already highlighted several times, the tricuspid pulse is to be considered as the normal pulse type. In Bertino, the normal carotid pulse provides the tracing represented in Fig. 12.1, line 1, recorded with the Marey tambour.

The highest pulsations correspond to the start of inspiration, which by the way was very superficial.

Here one sees very clearly that each individual pulsation consists of three elevations, of which the last two are almost of the same height. During and after inhalation of amyl nitrite (Fig. 12.1, line 2), the first elevation rises to a greater height and tends to dwindle, whereas the second descends to a lower point and becomes more distinct. Although we do not know the significance of these three elevations, we take stock of this fact and now go on to determine the modifications that take place in other body parts (e.g., the forearm).

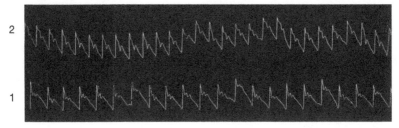

Figure 12.1 Bertino. Carotid pulse recorded with a Marey tambour applied to the neck. 1. In the normal state. 2. Under the influence of amyl nitrite.

In keeping with his profession as a farmer, Bertino's hands were so callous and the skin of his forearm so hard that he was little suited to more delicate investigations about the contour of the pulse.[1]

In order to provide a clear idea of the modifications brought forth by the inhalation of amyl nitrite in the cardiac impulse and in the pulsations of the forearm, I choose an example from a series of experiments that I conducted with my student, Mr. Rattone. For the sake of brevity, I omit the recording of the normal pulse and its modifications begun during the inhalation. The figure provided, Fig. 12.2, starts at the moment when the inhalation, which had lasted 30 seconds, was interrupted. A further portion of the original recording following upon the end of lines *A* and *C* of Fig. 12.2, lasting approximately 10 seconds, is again omitted. Then follows the portion of the pair of tracings represented in Fig. 12.3, in which the forearm pulsations increasingly approach the normal type, until at last, at the end of this leg, they have assumed more or less the same contour as prior to the inhalation. As we see, the normal pulse is also tricrotic.

In the normal state (end of line *C* in Fig. 12.3), the cardiac impulse recorded with the Marey cardiograph appears to be smaller than when under the influence of amyl nitrite.

With regard to the modification caused by this substance in the state of the vessels and consequently in the contour of the pulse, we see that the elevation *S* approaches the peak of the wave and nearly disappears in the instant of the most pronounced paralysis of the vessels, while the dicrotic elevation approaches the base of the wave and at last reaches its lowest point. The frequency of the

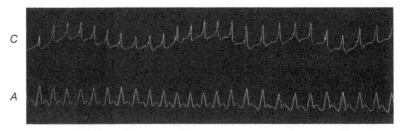

Figure 12.2 Rattone. Tracing of the cardiac impulse *C* and the forearm *A* under the influence of amyl nitrite.

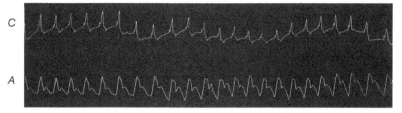

Figure 12.3 Continuation of the preceding tracing, recorded after a 10-minute interruption.

heartbeats becomes so great that this elevation no longer has time to express itself fully, and is finally (in the next to last pulse wave) missing entirely. This example may serve to prove how difficult it is to assess correctly the composition/quality of a pulsation when one does not have in front of one's eyes the complete sequence of the transformations of the pulse contour occurring within a certain period of time.

A factor not to be disregarded in the study of these modifications is the force of the heartbeats. By this I do not wish to imply that systole becomes more effective under the action of amyl nitrite and propels a greater quantity of blood into the circulation. Rather, if we take into account the fact that the vessels in the head and in the upper extremities are dilated, we must assume that the blood pressure is reduced (as has been demonstrated, by the way, in experiments on other animals).

Notwithstanding this, the impact of the heart against the chest wall is strengthened. It must be assumed that systole of the heart is more intense, but also that its diastolic expansion and the relaxation of its walls are greater. Of course, these are only assumptions; yet, since I have perceived several times that following heavy bleeding, when the animal is already dying and the blood pressure is weakened, the cardiac impulse strengthens, I must hold that the cardiac impulse does not constitute a decisive criterion for estimating the mechanical performance of systole.

The strengthening of the cardiac impulse is moreover not a constant phenomenon during inhalation of amyl nitrite, and the concomitant modifications of the contour of the heartbeat are almost imperceptible in comparison with the profound change experienced by the profile of each individual vascular pulsation both in the forearm and in the brain.

I have already referred to this subject in another treatise.[2]

In the cardiac tracing, the changes are less obvious with each time, and in the majority of cases one may say that aside from the increased frequency of contraction, there is no perceptible change in the cardiac impulse under the influence of amyl nitrite, while on the contrary, the contour of the forearm pulse has become quite different from the normal state.

If the modifications of the simultaneously recorded tracings of the forearm and of the heart differ both in their nature and in their shape and time period of occurrence, one easily understands how tentative (not to say, at this time already, **false**) the nowadays generally accepted teaching is, according to which one assumes that the characteristic signs of the pulse depend on events taking place in the heart.

It seems to me that much more befitting the facts is the interpretation I will develop in a study soon to be published. In it, I seek to demonstrate that the pulse observed in the brain, the forearm, and other body parts is not a reflection of the cardiac cycle, but a precise mirror image of the variations taking place in the vascular system. The heart determines the rhythm of the pulsations, while their contour is primarily dependent on the state of the vessels.

§. 12.3

A final remark I wish to make before the conclusion of this chapter relates to the fluctuations of the brain volume that I have observed under the influence of amyl nitrite. The paralysis of the blood vessels, which is produced by the vapors of this substance, can become much more extreme than was to be seen in tracings 39 to 42 of Plate 5.5. Once, when, instead of interrupting the inhalation after half a minute as in that experiment, I proceeded with it for over a minute until Bertino removed the cloth from his nose because he could not tolerate it any longer, I obtained the pulse tracing shown in Fig. 12.4.

To exclude the suspicion that perhaps the water contained in the Müllerian valves might by its fluctuations alter the contour of the pulse tracing, I employed in this experiment (as in all cases where it was important to study specifically the contour of the pulse) a simple thick-walled rubber tube, which connected the tubular attachment of the gutta percha plate A (woodcut, Fig. 2.1) with the recording barrel/tambour. A relief valve (clarinet), affixed to the tube, was vented from time to time to equalize the pressure in the levered barrel in the case of significant increases in brain volume. The cerebral pulse, which in the normal state (see the beginning of tracing 39, Plate 5.5) was subtricuspid and small, becomes very strong and bicuspid under the influence of amyl nitrite: the first elevation becomes imperceptible in that it blends with the heightened elevation S, while the dicrotic after-beat attains the height of the said elevation and the peak of the pulse wave thus obtains a bicuspid contour.

Now and then there appear, independent of the respiratory movements and of other known influences, great spontaneous undulations as in A and B of Fig. 12.4. I have seen a large undulation of this kind persist for 32 seconds.

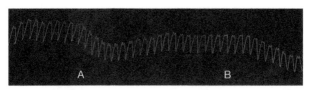

Figure 12.4 Bertino. Undulations of brain volume and changes of cerebral pulse during a forceful inhalation of amyl nitrite.

For the study of the modifications occurring in the pulse generally, it would be interesting to decide whether during the aforementioned experiments we have achieved through inhalation of amyl nitrite a complete paralysis of the vasculature in the brain and in the forearm. Unfortunately, I am not yet sufficiently acquainted with the topic to be able to make a definitive statement to that effect. Between contraction and normal tone, as well as between this and paralysis, there are intermediate states in the response of the arteries, veins, and capillaries that in physiology are unknown and with which I am at the very present occupied.

In order to be able to decide whether the undulations A and B in the tracing Fig. 12.4 obtained of Bertino with the use of amyl nitrite have been purely passive or partially active, I should also have recorded at the same time as the pulsations of the brain those of the forearm, or preferably of another body part (as, for example, the foot), upon which amyl nitrite reportedly does not exert any vessel-paralyzing influence. Unfortunately, I did not have enough time to conduct such comparative experiments; it therefore remains undecided whether, under the conditions considered previously, the cerebral vessels are to be regarded as completely paralyzed by the influence of amyl nitrite.

NOTES

1. Here I must regretfully recall a circumstance that nearly rendered impossible the execution of most of the experiments communicated in this work. On the first day, I had been given permission by the hospital that Bertino be allowed to come to my laboratory, and thus, at that time, I conducted with him a series of observations that are certainly among the most beautiful. Since then, however, the same permission was refused to me, even though the man was well and strolled around the garden all day long. I was therefore required to set up shop in a hospital room where I was continuously busy merely with putting together my devices or else with taking them apart. In such circumstances I could naturally not think about arranging everything with all the comfort necessary for such delicate experiments, and thus I had to refrain from many an interesting observation that I had intended to make. It is surely lamentable that in the largest hospital of a city such as Turin, scientific studies find so little encouragement. In this matter, one was, until recently, still in a deplorable state of dependence upon clerics and nuns, who are in command of the hospitals. [Trans.: In Mosso's earlier Italian manuscript, this final sentence is omitted, making his note more tersely diplomatic: ". . .È da deplorare che nell' ospedale primario di Torino fossero in allora così poco favorite le indagini scientifiche." No mention is made of hospital administrators.]
2. Mosso: *Die Diagnostik des Pulses.* Leipzig, 1879.

Anemia and Hyperemia of the Brain

§. 13.1

The fluctuations of the mental functions with decreasing or increasing blood flow to the brain form the subject of one of the most interesting studies with which the psychologist is able to engage experimentally, for there is no other way in which the intimate connection between the psychic and the material functions of the organism can be more visibly evidenced. It is enough to diminish the blood supply to the brain by just a small amount for consciousness to cease immediately. Should someone ask me which among all organic functions were tied most closely to any even minimal change of the metabolism, I would answer without hesitation: consciousness.

The molecular equilibrium in the organs, which are the seat of reason, is already deeply upset by influences that in no perceptible way disturb the functions of other body parts, because tissue metabolism in the brain takes place more actively and the makeup of constituent materials is more unstable. The higher value of psychic phenomena lies in the greater complexity of the events upon which they are based. One must also not be surprised if, as many others, I am inclined to consider the mind as the noblest expression of organic activity, simply because of all the manifestations of the organism, it most appears as servant of the metabolic substance.

The hemispheres of the cerebrum allow themselves to be affected so much by any influence that slows their nourishment but for one moment that the least reduction in the blood supply apportioned to them immediately abolishes consciousness.

Here is an observation on Bertino that is apt to put into glaring focus the unusual metabolic activity in the brain.

On September 29, at 1 o'clock in the afternoon, Dr. De Paoli and I agreed to conduct a few observations on cerebral anemia. To record the cerebral movements, we affixed an airtight gutta percha plate to the head of Bertino, and to make a simultaneous recording of the forearm pulse, we attached the hydrosphygmograph to his right arm. I explained to Bertino the purpose of our plan and asked him to pay very careful attention to everything that he felt in the course of the experiment so that he could tell us about it in detail afterward. I then sat down in front of him, applied the thumbs of each hand onto his respective carotids, and, while I observed the stylus of the recording barrel, compressed both vessels with gradually increasing strength until I saw the cerebral pulse cease, whereupon I immediately interrupted the compression. Bertino did not say anything. I then asked Dr. De Paoli, who stood behind the patient, to prepare for the compression of the carotids of our experimental subject. When my colleague told me that he felt both vessels pulsate beneath his fingers, I carved the symbol α onto the blackened paper of the kymograph (Fig. 13.1), and as soon as this had arrived at the styli, I motioned to the doctor to begin compression.

The first two pulsations rose in height, but the third was already smaller and the volume of the brain decreased rapidly. After the eighth systole, the pulse rate diminished significantly and the brain pulse became so small as to be barely visible. At the 14th pulsation i.e., after cerebral ischemia had been present for about 8 seconds, Bertino was seized by an epileptic fit. I looked at his face; he was pale, and his eyeballs were rolled upward. My colleague immediately released the carotids. As soon as Bertino reopened his eyes, almost surprised to find himself in this place and in this position, I attempted without delay to proceed with the recording of the pulsations; but the brain had experienced such a great increase in volume and the arm had moved so much that it became possible for me to resume recording of the brain pulse (tracing C' in Fig. 13.1) only 20 seconds after the initial appearance of the convulsions, and that of the forearm pulse about a minute later. When I saw that aside from the significant strengthening of the cerebral pulse there was nothing noteworthy, I interrupted the observation.

Bertino told us that during compression he experienced general darkness around him but did not have any unpleasant sensation. He spat on the floor, said that he felt some nausea, and soon after asked us to continue with the

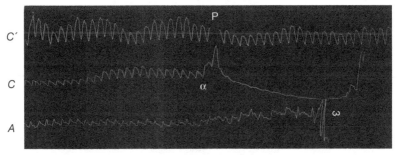

Figure 13.1 Bertino. Tracing of the forearm pulse A and of the cerebral pulse C, recorded at the same time as a generalized seizure caused by compression of the carotids. The compression of the carotid pulse lasted from α to ω. C' shows a continued tracing of the cerebral pulse, recorded 20 minutes after ceasing compression. At P, where a pulsation is missing, I had lifted the stylus so as not to distort the marked elevation of the tracing C underneath.

experiments. We remained surprised by his unusual indifference; however, since we had been more than a little frightened by that genuine epileptic seizure, during which the patient lost consciousness and raised high his hands balled up into fists, his face paled, and his eyes rolled upward, we did not have the courage either on that day or later to try another compression of the carotids.

The result of this experiment surprised me all the more since earlier on, I had compressed the carotids of Catherina X. and Johann Thron for a much longer period of time, almost until complete cessation of the cerebral pulsations, without there having been any such serious manifestations of brain anemia.

Fig. 13.2 shows two examples of carotid compression, which I had undertaken with Prof. Giacomini on Catherina X. In the upper line, compression of both carotids began at α and ended at ω; this was not as complete here as in the lower line, where it lasted approximately 30 seconds and the pulse disappeared nearly entirely, without there having occurred any threatening manifestations, let alone any convulsions. The woman retained full consciousness, even up to the last instant of compression, for she herself with her finger motioned to Prof. Giacomini, according to the previously given direction, to interrupt compression, which is what happened at point ω. The profile of the cerebral tracing in this case, compared to Bertino's (Fig. 13.1), reflects the different state of consciousness of both individuals. While in Bertino, in whom cerebral anemia provoked an epileptic fit, the cerebral tracing descended greatly with compression of the carotids, in Catherina X., it remained always horizontal with the same carotid compression, which leads to the assumption that in her case, the absence of any disturbance of consciousness rested not on a lesser receptivity of the psychic centers, but on the more complete compensation of the circulatory disturbance by the collateral tracts.

Conspicuous in this tracing is only the marked reinforcement of the cerebral pulsation after ceasing compression. I have already pointed out in a previous writing that when one simultaneously records the pulse of the brain and the forearm, this reinforcement of the former proves to be a purely local phenomenon. It is not controlled in the least by an increased force of the cardiac contractions, but rests merely on the relaxation of the vascular walls as a result of the interruption of the cerebral circulation. This paralysis of the vessels that comes about every time following an impairment of their nutrition is a phenomenon that can be demonstrated in the forearm with the greatest ease when one compresses with one's fingers the brachial artery and then allows the arm to fill freely with blood for some time.

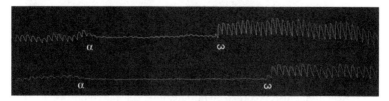

Figure 13.2 Catherina X. Modifications of the cerebral pulse during and after compression of the carotids, which lasted from α to ω.

I have at this moment before my eyes the entire series of experiments that I performed with compression of the carotid artery on Catherina X., Thron, and Bertino, and I compare the rise of the cerebral pulse after circulation has been restored with the analogous phenomenon that I noticed in the same three people and in the forearm of four others after compression of the brachial artery.

The difference is so great that it seems superfluous for me to add to the other already-published tracings, in order to be able to declare straight away as definite this fact: **that even to the most fleeting interruption of blood flow the cerebral vessels are much more sensitive than the vessels of the forearm.**

§. 13.2

In Chapter 4, during the discussion of the modifications that the blood circulation in the brain undergoes with stronger intellectual activity, such as with sensory and emotional impressions, I had only touched on the mechanical, hydraulic part of this complex question in taking into consideration only the passive variations, named so by me, that is, the variations of the brain volume resting on the contraction of the vessels of other body parts or on the changed rate and energy of the heartbeats.

Presently, we must examine those fluctuations of the blood circulation that stem from a change in innervation of elasticity of the cerebrovascular walls themselves, for the purpose of which we shall have to develop more comprehensively several considerations already indicated in Chapter 7, pp. 93–95, but only in a cursory way.

However, these local circulatory disturbances in the brain merit in-depth study all the more, since they come about not only in the open but also and just as well in the closed cranium.

One must recognize as justified the latter assertion, which might at first glance appear to be daring, after having seen in the next paragraph that the arterial blood vessels of the brain are able to contract and dilate at the expense of their concomitant veins. Furthermore, since it was known that in the closed skull, too, the cerebral blood vessels possess contractile walls and are equipped with appurtenant vasomotor nerves and centers, it was unthinkable at any rate that these systems would only exist not to accomplish anything.

Of all the body parts in which up to now I have studied the phenomena of the blood circulation, it is the brain where the variations in the state of the vessels are definitely the most frequent and the most prominent. Amid the uncommon unrest exhibited by the cerebral vessels, physiology is still incapable of distinguishing the reflex movements provoked by centripetal excitation of the vasomotor centers from the purely local phenomena, which rest upon chemical transfers in the province of the brain sections concerned. Yet, it can hardly be doubted that there are also phenomena of this latter category, for it is highly probable that the chemical transformation to which the material components of the brain are subject during the activity of the brain cells leads to the creation of products whose presence is enough to modify the elastic properties of the vessels supplying the substance of the brain.

The great variability in the state of the vascular walls reveals itself most conspicuously in the tracings obtained of the cerebral pulse, controlled by emotional influences. Tracings 1, 2, 3, and 4 AC of Plate 4.1 and tracing 6 RC of Plate 4.2 show us a very prominent and rapid relaxation of the cerebral vessels without there having been a contraction of those vessels preceding the increase in amplitude of the cerebral pulse and the increase in volume of the brain. The hyperemia of the brain, which sets in subsequent to emotional influences, is thus the compelling example of a relaxation of the blood vessels not preceded by a contraction of the same.

The fact that with increased mental activity, the augmentation of the brain volume coincides with a decrease in volume of the forearm could give room for the assumption that the dilatation of the blood vessels in the cerebral hemispheres reflects the cause for the lesser blood supply to the extremities. If one measures, according to the method indicated in § 5.1 (Chapter 2), the increase of cerebral volume during the most intense of the hyperemias/hyperemic states observed with increased mental activity and with emotional stimuli, one finds that the amount of blood accumulated in the brain equals much less than the volume decrease, as determined by plethysmography, of even one single forearm.

If, therefore, the assumption of a passive volume decrease of the forearm is excluded, which moreover also clearly follows from my observations about the profile of the forearm pulse during increased mental activity, according to which there is rather an active contraction of the forearm vessels, we must concede that the blood circulation in the brain is very often also modified by the activity of the particular vasomotor nerves of the cerebral vessels, and by the independent contraction or relaxation of the cerebral vessels produced in this way.

I have already indicated in Chapter 7 (see Figs. 7.1 and 7.2) how we may distinguish, simply by the contour of the pulse, passive volume decreases of the brain from a decrease based on active contraction of the cerebral vessels.

Let us review some tracings in which the increase of brain volume is entirely or partially controlled by independent modifications in the state of the cerebral vessels, independently from potential modifications in other body parts.

We have a nice example of such local modifications of the blood circulation in tracing 9 AC of Plate 4.2.

A few seconds after the symbol ℵ (which corresponds to the moment when I reprimanded Bertino), a very substantial rise in amplitude of the cerebral pulsations and of the volume of the brain sets in, and at the same time the forearm pulse becomes smaller (line 9 A). In this case, the hyperemia of the brain is not exclusively due to the contraction of the forearm vessels, but is to be attributed in part to the relaxation of the small arteries in the cerebral hemispheres. In the subsequent pair of lines 10 AC, we see that the hyperemia and the unusual amplitude of the brain pulsations persist (10 C), while the forearm vessels have now also, for their part, relaxed because of the secondary effect of emotion, as we learn from the contour and height of the forearm pulsations, the latter of which appears much greater in line 10 *A* than it had been at the onset of the emotional stimulus (line 9 *A*).

§. 13.3

An equally interesting phenomenon is the dilatation of the cerebral vessels that sets in some time after the conclusion of an intellectual task (as can be seen, for example, on Plate 5.4 at the end of line 30).

It is true that this subsequent vascular dilatation is not a constant phenomenon, but it is observed very frequently. As regards the significance, however, in all these cases, of the relaxation of the vascular walls, which is the basis for dilatation, it might be assumed that both increased mental activity and emotion are accompanied by an acceleration of metabolic consumption, the consequences of which are balanced by the augmented blood supply via the expanded blood vessels. The great vulnerability of the blood vessels and their tendency to dilate with every disturbance of metabolic balance represent one of the mechanisms by which the most important systems for the preservation of life are safeguarded.

At least, this is how I imagine the functional utility of these phenomena.

In the same sense as during or after increased metabolic consumption, the expansion of the vessels, which immediately opens the way for a more abundant blood supply, represents the most efficient factor through which, after a circulatory interruption, the nutritional and thus too the functional impairments of the brain and all other body parts are counterbalanced.

Earlier (in §. 13.1) I provided an example of the extraordinary rapidity with which cerebral metabolism takes place in showing how a transient circulatory obstruction gives rise immediately to serious functional disturbances on the part of this organ. The relationship of the psychic capacities to the phenomena of the blood circulation is so intimate that I did not hesitate to claim that the brain, among all organs, is least independent of the so-called material functions of the body. The sensory organs themselves are already infinitely superior to the brain in their ability to resist external agencies. We can produce an ischemia of the whole forearm by literally repressing blood from it with an elastic bandage, and we can maintain this state for 20 or even 25 minutes without the peripheral sensory devices of the nervous system losing their capacity to receive and conduct impressions of touch, warmth, and pain; with decrease of blood supply to the brain (for its complete interruption is not even necessary), however, a time period 300 times shorter is sufficient to abolish consciousness.

At the base of the skull there exists a vascular system that has no equal in the entire body. The joining of the vessels in the so-called circle of Willis—*circulus* (or more correctly *polygonum*) *Willisii*—results in the fact that the blood supply to the cerebral hemispheres never experiences a complete interruption, even if one of the four main arterial trunks becomes impassable. Moreover, the branches proceeding from this circle to nourish the brain are in their further course additionally equipped with rich continual anastomoses, and when there is any impairment of blood flow in one of these branches, all the remaining ones make up the shortfall of blood supply by collateral influx.

Although the reunion of the cerebral arteries in the circle of Willis represents a very simple and seemingly most effective anatomical arrangement, by means of which an immunity of the different parts of the brain against the consequences of a potential compression of the carotid or vertebral arteries would be expected, the compensation arising from this is nevertheless not perfect. In spite of this arrangement, which one would believe to be so effective and salutary for the integrity of the cerebral functions, every compensatory mechanism proves to be inadequate as soon as blood influx via one of the afferent arteries sinks below a certain level; this plainly demonstrates that the cerebral functions, which I therefore designate as the noblest of the body, require in their organs the most rapid metabolic exchange for the preservation of their integrity.

The great sensitivity of the brain to any influences impairing nutrition is even more obviously manifest in our previously mentioned experiment, inasmuch as 8 seconds was already enough for the blood supply, which persisted in both vertebral arteries (but was, of course, cut off in both carotids), to reveal itself as inadequate for the preservation of the metabolic needs of the phenomenon of consciousness.

Until now we have spoken of the impairment of blood replacement through direct obstruction of blood influx.

If we impair the renewal of blood in the brain through the obstruction of venous outflow, vascular tone is diminished and a similar effect as in ischemia is observed, even though to a much smaller degree. I refer to only one of the experiments conducted on Bertino for this purpose (see Plate 5.5, tracing 44).

The obstruction of venous outflow lasts from α to α and was performed by means of a band wound tightly around the neck, which impaired passage of blood in the jugular veins—that is, through downright strangulation. The Müller valves show us by their oscillations the number of air bubbles entering into and leaving the apparatus. If we compare the brain pulsations before and after strangulation, we see that they become more ample afterward. Through simultaneous recording of the forearm pulse, I could be certain that this phenomenon was based solely on the localized decrease of vascular tone, for there was a lack of any participation in the forearm.

Since I started my investigations of the blood circulation in the human brain, I have had to persuade myself that the amount of blood inside the skull can increase significantly without critical perturbations of the mental functions arising.

If venous flow is simply dammed up, everyone easily understands that this kind of circulatory disturbance is of lesser import for the nourishment of the brain. But this matter becomes of much greater significance in the theory nowadays generally accepted by physiologists about the nature of cerebral phenomena and their dependence on blood circulation, when we see that even a very substantial arterial hyperemia of the brain can take place without there being the slightest alteration of intellectual functions.

Here is where the case described in the previous chapter (about the effect of amyl nitrite) belongs, in which we see the cerebral circulation accelerate markedly, the brain volume increase, and the arteries dilate, without any abnormal occurrence in the psychic condition except for the sensation of warmth of the facial skin.

It seems to me that the lack of relationship between the increase of blood quantity contained within the skull and mental activity is founded on the fact that regarding the latter, it is not the blood content of the brain that is important, but rather that it is necessary for the blood in the psychic centers to flow under heightened pressure when in these structures the events of metabolism and along with them the functional performances should be incited more vigorously. If the cerebral vessels expand due to an action inducing vascular paralysis, as happens during inhalations of amyl nitrite, we may assume that in spite of the greater blood filling of the arterial vessels in the brain, the utility of the latter for functional operations is nil because blood pressure is thereby diminished. It is true that with strengthened cerebral activity, the volume increase observed by us may be lesser, but blood circulation is nevertheless more active, in that the blood streams through the cerebral vessels under increased pressure and with greater velocity. If one inclines the head forward, venous obstruction takes place, as I have also had occasion to confirm by direct observations on Bertino and Catherina X. (I do not reproduce the tracings concerned since they are of no particular interest.)

Indeed, the circulatory disturbance arising under such circumstances can lead, as we know, to dizziness, visual blurring, and even more serious accidents in many people.

Concerning the Blood Circulation Inside the Intact Skull

§. 14.1

In the introduction to this book, I described the history of the still controversial question about the blood circulation in the intact skull and attempted a critical illumination thereof. In the interest of conciseness, I believe I may be permitted here to refrain from repeating the observations developed there.

In the present chapter, we will discuss this question on the basis of our own investigations.

Because the skull represents an inflexible and overall closed capsule, I had the idea that the venous blood inside might flow under a higher pressure because here, in addition to the *vis a tergo*, there is another force not coming to the fore in other body parts, namely, the pulsatile expansion of the arteries. The wave of blood penetrating into the skull causes a diastole of all brain arteries, and this expansion of the arterial vascular tree generated by the force of the cardiac systole creates pressure on the cerebral veins so that with every pulsation, the venous blood undergoes a thrust, which propels it into the cranial venous sinuses with a pressure higher than that which would be the case only with the *vis a tergo*.

The experiment confirmed the validity of this assumption.

I trephined the skull of dogs at the midline, exposed the sinus longitudinalis, and opened it without entering the meningeal space so that the experimental results were not contaminated by the pressure of the cephaloarachnoid fluid. I established the connection of the cerebral sinus with a manometer by means of a metallic tube screwed tightly into the cranial wall of the same diameter as the trephining crown used to open the skull. In order to obtain an exact measure of the differences that the cranial veins present compared to those of other body parts where the pressure is higher, I used the differential manometer and combined the blood pressure of the crural vein with that of the cerebral sinus.

Here is a brief list of the data of one of these experiments.

I chose a large dog, anaesthetized him with chloroform, and then prepared the crural vein, into which I inserted a cannula. From there a tube went to the differential mercury manometer. I then trephined the skull near the brain, in the free corner between the origination of the masseters. The bone here was very thick. I carefully detached the section of bone, waited until venous bleeding from the diploe stopped, and then screwed in the slightly cone-shaped tube. With a small knife I incised the sinus that lay in the center of the skull opening. A strong venous hemorrhage ensued and blood spurted from the tube. I immediately established the connection with the second leg of the differential manometer and found that the blood pressure in the cranial sinus was 3 cm higher than that in the crural vein. The animal at this moment was deeply anesthetized. To the extent that it awakened from this and the expiratory movements strengthened, the difference also rose, until the excess pressure on the part of the skull reached 6 cm.

In order to simplify the experiment, I first took the precaution to bring the animal and the manometer into such a position that the tube inserted into the skull, the cannula of the crural vein, and the level of mercury in both legs of the manometer were placed on a horizontal level; I kept the leg suspended in such a way that its circulation remained unobstructed.

I again anesthetized the dog with chloroform, and the difference between the amount of pressure in the sinus and in the crural vein decreased. At the moment that anesthesia had set in and breathing had become very superficial, the cranial blood pressure was still 1 cm higher than the pressure in the crural vein. I let the anesthesia lapse, and when the pressure differential had again risen to 55 mm, I killed the animal by exsanguination.

The autopsy revealed that within the diploe, two sturdy veins emptied near the vicinity of the trephining opening. There was no hemorrhage in the brain. The cut severed only the wall of the sinus without penetrating into the meningeal space.

––––––––––––––––

In order to determine the exact amount of pressure of the venous blood in the skull, I used a simple mercury manometer, which I connected to the frontal portion of the longitudinal sinus in the manner indicated earlier. During the time in which the animal was deeply anesthetized, the manometer recorded a pressure of 70 to 80 mm; later, the pressure rose gradually up to 100 to 110 mm. After determining this value for the pressure amount in the longitudinal sinus of the skull, I killed the animal by injury of the medulla oblongata. I lowered an awl into the vertebral cavity, and a very strong increase of the pressure in the cranial veins was shown: the mercury column of the manometer rose to 160 mm and showed strong pulsations that corresponded to the slow but powerful contractions of the heart.

Autopsy undertaken immediately after death revealed that during the incision of the sinus, the point of the knife had also breached its posterior wall and had penetrated into the meningeal space, where a blood clot was found. However, I could not discover any injury of either the brain or its vessels.

On the basis of these results, still to be confirmed by further experiments, I believe I can state that **venous blood flow inside the skull takes place under a higher pressure than in any other part of the body in which it has been measured up to now.**

§. 14.2

In the course of these manometric measurements, I had (as I mentioned during the last experiment) made the observation that the mercury column showed rhythmic rises, which temporally coincided with the cardiac contractions.

Having been led in this way to the traces of a venous pulse in the cranial sinuses, I found that this idea is not totally new, for H. Berthold,[1] who undertook a series of experiments to explain the venous pulse in the fundus of the eye, already reported that in a dog, after ligation of the common jugular vein, he saw the blood spurt forth from the injured interior jugular vein in a rhythmically broken up jet, as that from an artery.

This observation is quite correct, and I was able to confirm the fact and represent it graphically both in the internal jugular vein (into which, for this purpose, I introduced a cannula at its point of exit from the skull) and in the sinuses according to the previously mentioned procedure (by means of a metallic tube bored into the skull and plunged directly into a venous sinus). To those who might wish to repeat the experiment, I particularly recommend the latter procedure as being the easier one. Indeed, it would be even better to place the trephining crown in the occipital region and thus attain the location of the confluence of the cerebral sinuses (*torcular herophili*).

For the graphic representation of these pulsations, it is more advisable to use instead of a mercury manometer a levered tambour, which one fills with a solution of sodium carbonate and to which, right after the incision of the anterior wall of the sinus, one connects the metallic tube inserted into the cranial wall. During the incision of the sinus, one must be careful not to strike through its posterior wall into the meningeal space. The tambour that I used had a diameter of 20 mm and was covered with a fairly sturdy elastic membrane. The oscillations of the membrane were communicated to the lever resting against its center and transcribed onto a blackened cylinder.

The tracing here reproduced (Fig. 14.1) was obtained with the *sinus longitudinalis* following this procedure. The autopsy showed that the incision was restricted to the anterior wall of the sinus and did not penetrate into the meningeal space, for there was neither blood clot nor injection at the corresponding site of the brain surface.

Tracing 1 represents the pulse of the longitudinal sinus during deep chloroform anesthesia of the experimental animal (dog). Breathing was very shallow. Tracing 2 similarly refers to the pulse of the longitudinal sinus but was recorded a few minutes later, when respiration became somewhat deeper than in the normal state after the effect of the chloroform had worn off. Tracing 3 is the pulse of the left carotid. It is recorded immediately after tracing 2, and in fact with the same apparatus as the two preceding ones, but here the elastic membrane of the recording tambour was made less flexible by winding an elastic rubber thread several times around it. The anacrotic contour of the carotid pulse must be emphasized, which is expressed by a slight curve of the ascending leg of almost every individual pulse wave.

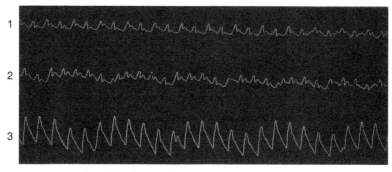

Figure 14.1 Dog. Pulse of the *longitudinal sinus* during (1) and after (2) deep chloroform anesthesia, together with the pulse of the left carotid (3) recorded just after the second sinus tracing.

As one can see in this tracing, the venous blood inside the skull, like the arterial blood, is engaged in pulsatile movement. The pulse is dicrotic and often tricrotic, and the tracing shows respiratory fluctuations very similar to those we have found in all arteries of the body.

On the basis of these experiments, then, it seems to me fully demonstrated that the arterial blood flow in the brain can experience, without hindrance, even in the closed skull, all those variations it has presented to us in other body parts. With every diastole of the arteries there occurs a systole of the veins, which leave room for the blood volume penetrating into the brain. And for the respiratory oscillations, it is also the venous vascular trunk that, through the oscillations of the blood contained within it, makes possible the alternating expansion and contraction of the arterial vascular trunk.

My experiments have thus furnished a factual basis for the assumption of a mechanism that had already been foreseen, albeit only on theoretical grounds, by Lorry and Cappie (see p. 15).

However, we assert on the basis of our observations that in the closed skull, there is a mechanism that takes place either exclusively or along with others, but in any case predominantly, through which not just the amount of blood contained in the skull varies, but also its distribution to the arteries, capillaries, and veins. The wave of blood entering into the arterial flow displaces a corresponding amount of blood from the veins and imparts to the venous bloodstream a pulsatile movement very similar to that taking place in the arteries.

This mechanism explains the consequences arising from the fact that the cranial veins are not equipped with valves and empty into rigidly walled sinuses.

The veins of the abdominal cavity, too, lack valves, and I think it is very probable that the functions of these, up to this day unexplained, anatomical characteristics are the same for both body cavities. If the blood were not able to back up during the pressure swings produced in the abdominal cavity by the respiratory movements, but were compelled by valves attached to the venous walls to stream into the liver with the full force of the intra-abdominal pressure, these powerful impulses would have, I believe, detrimental consequences for the portal system and for the functions of the liver.

It is probable that in the skull, the lack of venous valves results in promoting the fluctuations of the blood circulation in the brain, for the space that the arteries leave through their contraction is easily occupied by the backing up of venous blood, which would not be possible in the presence of valves.

The continual changes in volume, to which the brain is subjected because of the arterial diastole and the respiratory movements, even the very weight of the organ itself during different positions of the head, could easily produce obstacles to venous outflow if the great efferent trunks were not protected against such damaging influences by the support of the anatomical conditions. This favorable anatomic mechanism is known to consist of the small venous branches emptying into stiffly walled sinuses. The inflexibility of these canals constitutes the highly simple arrangement upon which rests the securing of the blood circulation in the brain, otherwise so difficult to explain, so that arteries and capillaries can expand and narrow without hindrance or disadvantage while the organ is enclosed inside a rigid bony capsule that shields it against external harm.

The ideas that I already developed in the chapter about the nature of sleep relieve me of further considerations about the utility of the anatomic conditions to which I have just directed readers' attention. Presuming the need for all organisms to adapt to external circumstances and to adjust the functions of their organs in a way most conducive to preserve life, we may also, for brevity's sake, use the traditional teleologic terminology and call purpose that which is the result of a factual but unconscious striving. Yet it might be more appropriate not to use conventional expressions, which can lead to tendentious misinterpretations.

NOTES

1. H. Berthold: *Zur Blutcirculation in geschlossenen Höhlen*. Centralblatt für die medicinischen Wissenschaften, 1879, n. 43.

Investigations Into the Movements of the Cerebrospinal Fluid

§. 15.1

Until the present it has been frequently assumed that the displacements of the cerebrospinal fluid give, within certain limits, free play to the brain for volume fluctuations. It can now be easily demonstrated that this theory of the movements of the arachnoid fluid is partially incorrect. The great resistances, which said fluid would have to overcome during its passage from the skull into the vertebral canal and vice versa, let us assume a priori that it undergoes no such change of location with the more rapid volume fluctuations, pulsations, and even respiratory oscillations of the brain, for with these the mechanism indicated on pp. 210 to 211 may take place much more easily.

If we connect a manometer with the cerebrospinal fluid contained within the vertebral canal or if we observe the membrana obturatoria posterior and see in both cases oscillations that correspond to the phases of respiration, this does not then demonstrate that a crossing of cerebrospinal fluid from the skull to the vertebral canal and vice versa is taking place. I have already shown in another writing[1] that the conclusions Magendie, Ecker, and Richet drew from similar observations in favor of the presumed passage were altogether gratuitous. Under such conditions, one may only conclude that the pressure under which the cerebrospinal fluid remains decreases in inspiration and increases in expiration.

My experiments regarding this question allow me to refute most emphatically that the cerebrospinal fluid crosses from one cavity into the next with every pulsation; we will see why one must reject such a transition even in the case of stronger but slower changes in volume, which take place in the nervous centers as a result of the respiratory movements.

I believe I need hardly note that I do not at all intend to reject the connection between the subarachnoid spaces of the spinal cord and those of the brain.

Salathé,[2] who conducted a series of experiments on cerebral movements in Prof. Marey's laboratory, trephined areas of the skull and of the vertebral column respectively and attached a recording apparatus to each borehole. He found that the two tracings obtained showed pulsations as well as respiratory oscillations and were parallel in their course, and specifically that with expiration the cerebrospinal fluid rose, and with inspiration it sank simultaneously in both devices.

I repeated this experiment with a minor modification, and, as one will see in the next section, obtained with respect to the occurrence of said facts only slightly deviating results. However, a few new data that I had occasion to determine here do not permit me any longer to affirm the view that I myself had defended in my earlier studies, and that Salathé (like Richet and others) believed he must, on the basis of his experiments, maintain: the view that, since the brain, with each cardiac systole, receives more blood than the spinal cord, a corresponding amount of cerebrospinal fluid must at the same time flow from the cranial cavity into the vertebral canal; that the very same takes place with expiration and with muscle exertion, because here, too, the intracranial vessels receive more blood than the spinal cord; but that, during cardiac diastole, inspiration, and muscular relaxation, the cerebrospinal fluid flows back again from the spinal canal into the skull.

In spite of all pertinent theoretical considerations and investigations, until now there was no obvious experimental proof that under normal circumstances such a transit flow of the cerebrospinal fluid truly took place.

To solve this question, I have conducted experiments on a 6-month-old child afflicted with spina bifida for one part and on dogs for the other, which here I want to recollect briefly.

§. 15.2

I inserted a tube in the curvature of the loin rib of a dog and, like Salathé, connected the cerebrospinal fluid to a recording apparatus in the manner described previously (§14.1). I trephined another hole into the cranial wall with the trepan without injuring the superior crescent-shaped sinus, and here, too, with an apparatus very similar to the first, recorded the movements of the cerebrospinal fluid. The pulsations of the vertebral column were barely visible. I gradually increased the resistance of the elastic membrane at the head tambour by wrapping it with a thin rubber thread, which hindered the rising motion of the elastic membrane and of the aluminum plate serving as support for the lever. The excursions of the loin tambour did not therefore increase. I wound more threading around the head tambour until at the skull all pulsations of the cerebrospinal fluid stopped. In the vertebral column, the pulsations remained equal and barely visible.

On the basis of this experiment, one may well assume that during the pulsations of the brain, there is really no transmission of the cerebrospinal fluid into the spinal canal, which takes place. For the contrary to be accepted, the pulsations of the fluid in the spinal canal would have to become more ample under the conditions of our experiment, if the cerebral pulse cannot become manifest. However, this does not stand our test. This is due to the role played herein by the veins, which empty under a far lower pressure than that required for displacing suddenly the cerebrospinal fluid from the skull into the spinal canal.

After having persuaded myself that after each inspiration the column of fluid moved toward the cranial cavity as well as toward the spinal canal, I interrupted the external connection of the loin opening (i.e., with a pipette). If at this moment there truly existed such a strong aspiration from the cranial cavity that it would be able to exert a visible effect onto the cerebrospinal fluid in the lumbar area, there would have to now be the production of a stronger backflow of the fluid column toward the skull, and that was just not the case. The respiratory oscillations in the skull cavity remained constant. And similarly, the much smaller amplitude of the spinal respiratory fluctuations remained unchanged when the skull opening was sealed.

The negative result of this experiment is sufficient to refute Richet's statement, which asserts the following: "*à chaque inspiration le liquide remonte dans la cavité encéphalique qui le repompe*"[3] [Trans.: "With each inspiration the fluid rises back up into the cerebral cavity, which pumps it out again"]. The pressure decrease in the spinal canal during inspiration is evidently not based on an aspiration, which pulls the cerebrospinal fluid into the cranial cavity, because, then, through the removal of the communication with the horizontal tube attached in the lumbar region, we would certainly have increased the obstacles to the movement of the cerebrospinal fluid through the spinal canal toward the skull, and then the backflow of the fluid in the horizontal tube of the skull would have had to become stronger. The absence of such a strengthening is proof that the pressure decrease in the spinal canal and the pressure decrease in the skull cavity are two localized phenomena, independent of one another, quite analogous to the pressure decrease that takes place in the cylinder of the plethysmograph wherein we have enclosed the forearm.

If one had considered only for a moment the wealth of veins of the brain, the extreme capacity of these veins to dilate, and the insignificance of the volume changes occurring with the respiratory fluctuations, one would never have been able to conceive of the hypothesis that a negative pressure of sufficient force could be produced in the brain to raise a column of fluid such as that of the spinal subarachnoid space.

§. 15.3

The observations I had occasion to conduct in conjunction with Prof. S. Fubini in a case of spina bifida in a human subject led to essentially congruent results.

The case was that of a 6-month-old girl, who presented with a tumor in the lumbar region the size of a hen's egg, which communicated directly with the spinal canal and was easily emptied into it by pressure. The skin at the peak of the swelling was so thin that the liquid content shimmered through and rupture was feared to occur at any moment. We hurried, therefore, to seize this exceedingly favorable opportunity to investigate the movements of the cerebrospinal fluid in man, and we undertook a series of experiments to determine whether any pulsatile movement could be perceived in the tumor.

The first apparatus we used for this purpose consisted of a small gutta-percha hat, the floor (peak) of which covered the entire swelling while sealing its base hermetically with clasps fastened to the surrounding skin. A small glass tube was inserted into the floor of the hat, which connected the air contained in the space between the surface of the tumor and the interior surface of the hat with a Marey *tambour régistrateur*. The tracings we obtained while the child lay still on her stomach and slept showed us that the quiet and shallow breathing exerted an already noticeable influence on the volume of the tumor; however, we were unable to perceive any pulsations synchronous with the heartbeat.

We then tried to fill the space between the tumor and the gutta-percha hat with fluid and to replace the recording apparatus with a thin, horizontal pipette. Yet with this procedure, too, there were no pulsations manifest in the tumor: the fluctuations of the column of fluid in the pipette corresponded merely to the respiratory movements and we saw, as before, that after each inspiration there followed a decrease in volume, and with each expiration an increase in the volume, of the swelling.

After these first experiments for the discovery of a pulse movement in the tumor synchronous with the heartbeat had proved unsuccessful, we tried another method. That is, we attempted to augment the oscillations of the skin at the peak of the swelling by directly applying a lever to the location where this skin appeared to be most markedly thinned out. After first spreading a little oil on the tumor, we molded its shape with gypsum mixed with tepid water. We found after filling this plaster cast with water that its volumetric content (i.e., the volume of the tumor) at the moment of measurement approximated 14 cm^3. Then we drilled a round hole into the tip of the mold, in which, when we repositioned the plaster mold, the tip of the tumor was to lie freely exposed. At the rim of this 1-cm opening we attached a light, small lever 20 cm in length, to which we affixed a thin crossbar (exactly at a right angle to the lever bar) directly next to the support point. The tip of the latter was furthermore equipped with a small ball of wax, which was intended to rest on the peak of the swelling and, after previous warming, to adhere lightly to it. In this way, the plaster mold provided firm support to the lever, and since its interior surface was covered with grease, the movements of expansion and contraction of the tumor were concentrated in the exposed tip, which was in contact with the lever. Yet with this method, too, we only perceived very distinct respiratory fluctuations, at the height of which there were indeed smaller oscillations, but we were unable to determine with certainty whether each of these corresponded to the rhythm of the heartbeat. The exceedingly propitious conditions under which we conducted these observations as well as the great care we took in executing them lend undeniable weight to these negative results, and thus at a minimum justify the conclusion that **with spina bifida, pulsatile movement of the tumor, synchronous with the heartbeat, can be quite absent even under conditions seemingly favorable to its perception.**

Furthermore, if the cerebrospinal fluid could easily flow from the cranial cavity into the spinal cavity, pulsations of the tumor should have set in at least at the

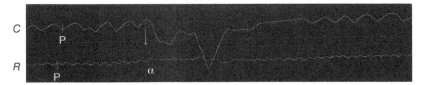

Figure 15.1 Behavior of the fontanel pulse *C* in a child with spina bifida, initially with untouched lumbar tumor, then during its compression lasting a few seconds (↓α). *R*, respiratory tracing.

point when we positioned the child in such a way that her head was lower than the level of the lumbar region. Yet even in this case, there was in the tumor no perceptible trace of pulsations synchronous with the heartbeat.

Much more interesting with regard to the topic discussed in this chapter are the experiments we conducted in the child with spina bifida regarding the behavior of the fontanel pulse with compression of the lumbar swelling. A Marey tambour, which recorded the pulse graphically, was applied to the anterior fontanel. Since the movements of the child might otherwise have distorted the tracings, all experiments here described were conducted during sleep. A Marey pneumograph applied to the thorax recorded the respiratory movements (Fig. 15.1, tracing *R*) while the child lay sleeping on her abdomen.

At point ↓α, I suddenly grasped the swelling with my fingers and compressed it so that more than half of its fluid content was driven back into the spinal cavity. The fontanel pulse weakened. A prolonged and deep inspiration ensued. The child awoke as if frightened and cried for a while. The nurse offered her breast to the child, and the child started sucking immediately and then fell asleep again. In this as well as in earlier experiments, I observed the child during compression, and as soon as I saw that she stirred and awakened, I interrupted the compression, whereupon the tumor immediately regained its previous volume.

The experiment was repeated on several days and each time the volume increase of the brain proved to be very slight, barely worth mentioning, even if through compression 10 or 12 cm³ of fluid were pushed back into the spinal cavity. For example, in the case represented in Fig. 15.2, the swelling had been compressed to the point of disappearance.

Regarding the interpretation of this phenomenon, we had repeatedly observed that during compression of the swelling in the lumbar region the brain pulse in the fontanel waned, and therefore the supposition emerged in us that the pressure of the fluid within the spinal canal might possibly lead to arrest of the heartbeat. Our first inquiries pertaining to this regarding the radial pulse and the apical cardiac impulse had equivocal results, and we therefore took recourse to auscultation. We then found that with increased pressure of the cerebrospinal fluid, while the cardiac thrusts did not stop entirely, they nevertheless weakened.

Thus, there was present, if not complete arrest, an inhibition of cardiac activity. After discontinuing compression, one noticed a slight decrease of the pulse rate in comparison to the original one, which indicated an increase of cardiac contractions.

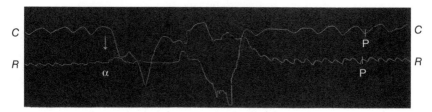

Figure 15.2 Behavior of the fontanel pulse *C* and the respiratory movements *R* in the same child, initially with untouched lumbar tumor, later during firmer compression of the same (↓α), during which about 10 or 12 cm³ of fluid was pushed back into the spinal cavity.

Now one might think that both the transient inhibition of cardiac activity and the subsequent strengthening and slowing of cardiac contractions are causally related to the rise of the fontanel tracing and the increase of its individual pulsations noticed after discontinuing compression of the tumor. We have seen in previously discussed experiments that the vessels of the brain surpass in sensitivity those of other organs inasmuch as after localized decelerations of the circulation, a subsequent expansion sets in more easily and to a prominent degree within them. It can hardly be doubted that such is also the case when the slowing of the blood circulation in the cerebral vessels is related to a disturbance in the general circulation.

Yet another, no less plausible assumption would be that a sensory excitation caused by sudden compression of the swelling resulted in relaxation of the frontal vessels, such as we have observed multiple times after the effect of emotional stimuli (see Chapter 4).

Finally, as regards the issue of the passage of the cerebrospinal fluid from the spinal cavity into the skull and vice versa, the two experiments described just now demonstrate in any case that there can be no question of an **easy** transit of this kind, since during the second experiment, where 10 or 12 cm³ of fluid had been pushed back into the spinal cavity with some force, the skin over the anterior fontanel rose only very slightly during the compression.

The event of a more pronounced rise at the fontanels can thus be interpreted only in this way, and not by any deep inspiration caused by the compression of the swelling: insofar as the *liquor cerebrospinalis* flowed easily into the skull, there should have occurred, already at the first moment of compression and still before the coming about of the deep inspiration—in fact, even at its start—a much later rise of the fontanel tracing.

NOTES

1. Mosso: *Introduzione ad una serie di esperienze su I movimenti del cervello nell' uomo.* Archivio per le scienze mediche, I, fasc. 2, 1876, p. 17.
2. Salathé: *Recherches sur les mouvements du cerveau.* Paris, 1877, p. 111.
3. Richet: Anatomie medico-chirurgicale, 1866, p. 53.

Thron, Giovanni
  brain studies on, 33, 37–38, 44
  carotid compression studies on,
      180–181
  cerebral pulse variations, 52–53, 69
  sleep studies on, 74, 76–79, 101, 104–105
Traube, M., 98, 163
Tricuspid pulse configuration
  blood vessel condition and, 57–62
  food intake effect on, 55
  overview, 49–52

Unconscious activity, doctrine of, 92

Vascular tone, 131
Vertigo, 125, 185
Vesalius (ancient Greece and Rome), 8
Vessels. *See* Blood vessels
Visual blurring, 185
Vitalist ideas, 15

Waking up, cerebral volume when, 76,
      89, 95

Zoroaster (ancient Greece and Rome), 7